Neuropathic Pain

What Do I Do Now? — Pain Medicine

SERIES EDITORS

Mark P. Jensen and Lynn R. Webster

PUBLISHED AND FORTHCOMING TITLES

Neuropathic Pain

Edited by
Nadine Attal and Didier Bouhassira
Hôpital Ambroise Paré, Boulogne-Billancourt, France, and UVSQ
Paris-Saclay University, Versailles, France

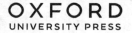

OXFORD
UNIVERSITY PRESS

OXFORD
UNIVERSITY PRESS

Oxford University Press is a department of the University of Oxford. It furthers
the University's objective of excellence in research, scholarship, and education
by publishing worldwide. Oxford is a registered trademark of Oxford University
Press in the UK and certain other countries.

Published in the United States of America by Oxford University Press
198 Madison Avenue, New York, NY 10016, United States of America.

Library of Congress Cataloging-in-Publication Data
Names: Attal, N., author, editor. | Bouhassira, Didier, author, editor.
Title: Neuropathic pain / Nadine Attal, Didier Bouhassira.
Other titles: What do I do now?. Pain medicine
Description: New York : Oxford University Press, [2023] |
Series: What do I do now?. Pain medicine |
Includes bibliographical references and index.
Identifiers: LCCN 2022040747 (print) | LCCN 2022040748 (ebook) |
ISBN 9780197616345 (paperback) | ISBN 9780197616369 (epub) |
ISBN 9780197616376 (online)
Subjects: MESH: Neuralgia—diagnosis | Neuralgia—therapy | Case Reports
Classification: LCC RC412 (print) | LCC RC412 (ebook) | NLM WL 544 |
DDC 616.8—dc23/eng/20221206
LC record available at https://lccn.loc.gov/2022040747
LC ebook record available at https://lccn.loc.gov/2022040748

DOI: 10.1093/med/9780197616345.001.0001

Printed by Marquis, Canada

Contents

SECTION 2 COMMON THERAPEUTIC OPTIONS

Contributors

Charles Argoff, MD
Professor of Neurology
Director, Division of Chronic Pain
Management
Associate Program Director, Pain
Medicine Fellowship
Department of Anesthesiology
Albany Medical Center
Albany, NY, USA

Nadine Attal, MD, PhD
Professor of Therapeutics and Pain
Medicine
Head of Pain Clinical Center
INSERM U 987 and UVSQ Paris
Saclay University
Boulogne Billancourt, France

Ralf Baron, Dr Med
Professor of Neurology
Head of Division of Neurological
Pain Research and Therapy
Head of Division of Neurological
Pain Research and Therapy
Department of Neurology
University Hospital
Schleswig-Holstein
Kiel, Germany

David LH Bennett, MB, PhD
Professor of Neurology
Nuffield Department of Clinical
Neuroscience
University of Oxford
Oxford, UK

Ravneet Bhullar
Associate Professor of
Anesthesiology
Director of the Division of Chronic
Pain Management
Associate Program Director
Chronic Pain Fellowship
Department of Anesthesiology
Albany Medical Center
Albany, NY, USA

Didier Bouhassira
INSERM Research Director
Head of INSERM U 987 Unit
Ambroise Paré Hospital, APHP
UVSQ Paris-Saclay University
Versailles, France

**Daniel Ciampi de Andrade,
MD, PhD**
Professor of Neurology
Health Science and Technology
Faculty of Medicine
Center for Neuroplasticity and
Pain, Aalborg Universitet
Aalborg, Denmark

Gianfranco de Stefano, MD, PhD
Department of Human
Neuroscience
Sapienza University
Rome, Italy

Nanna Brix Finnerup, MD, Dr MedSc
Professor of Neuropathic Pain
Research
Department of Clinical Medicine
Danish Pain Research Center
Aarhus University
Aarhus, Denmark

Eleonora Galosi
Department of Human
Neuroscience
Sapienza University
Rome, Italy

Janne Gierthmühlen MD PhD
Professor of Neurology and Pain
Medicine
Chief of Pain Care Department
Department of Anesthesiology,
Intensive Care Medicine and Pain
University Hospital
Schleswig-Holstein
Kiel, Germany

Sandra Sif Gylfadottir MD
Associate Professor
Department of Neurology and
Department of Clinical Medicine
Danish PainResearch Center
Aarhus University Hospital and
Aarhus University
Aarhus, Denmark

Dilara Kersebaum, MD
Resident
Division of Neurological Pain
Research and Therapy
Department of Neurology
University Hospital
Schleswig-Holstein
Kiel, Germany

Xavier Moisset, MD, PhD
Professor
Department of Neurology
NeuroDol
Université Clermont
Auvergne, CHU de Clermont
Ferrand, Inserm
Clermont Ferrand, France

Benjamin Portal, MD
Department of Neurology
Albany Medical Center
Albany, NY, USA

Michael C. Rowbotham, MD
Adjunct Professor of Anesthesia
and Emeritus Professor of
Neurology, UCSF
Attending Physician, UCSF Pain
Management Center
Department of Anesthesia
University of California
San Francisco, School of Medicine
San Francisco, CA, USA

Manon Sendel, MD
Resident
Division of Neuropathic Pain
Research and Therapy
Department of Neurology
University Hospital
Schleswig-Holstein
Kiel, Germany

**Andreas Themistocleous,
MBChB, PhD, FCP(SA), MRCP**
Clinical Lecturer in
Neurophysiology
Nuffield Department of Clinical
Neurosciences
University of Oxford
Oxford, UK

Grégory Tosti
Centre d'Evaluation et Traitement
de la Douleur
Hôpital Ambroise Paré
Boulogne-Billancourt, France

Anne-Priscille Trouvin, MD
Clinical Lecturer in Therapeutics
and Pain Medicine
Department of Pain Medicine
Cochin University Hospital—
Université Paris Cité
Paris, France

Andrea Truini, MD
Professor of Neurology
Department of Human
Neuroscience
Sapienza University
Rome, Italy

Lise Ventzel, PhD
Department of Oncology
Vejle Hospital, University Hospital
of Southern Denmark
Lillebaelt Hospital Vejle, University
Hospital of Southern Denmark
Vejle, Denmark

Clinical Cases, Diagnosis, and Management

1   Is This Neuropathic Pain?

Nadine Attal and Didier Bouhassira

A 66-year-old man with a 3-year history of type II
diabetes treated by metformin visits you because of
pain involving the lower limbs. His lower limb pain
appeared 18 months ago and is rated as severe on
a 0–10 numerical rating scale (7/10). He states that
his pain is aggravated by stress and contact with
sheets at night, and it causes insomnia. Pain involves
the plantar surface and dorsum of the feet, extends
to the ankles, and is bilateral and symmetric. It is
mainly described as burning, associated with electric
shocks, tingling, pins and needles, and numbness.
Neurological examination shows decreased sensation
to pinprick and pain induced by brushing of the feet,
no motor impairment, no abnormal reflexes and
normal vibration sense. Blood tests are within normal
ranges except for hyperglycemia and a high low-
density lipoprotein cholesterol level. Hemoglobin A1C
level is 10%.

What do you do now?

This patient with uncontrolled type II diabetes reports chronic pain at the feet. In the context of diabetes, pain at the lower limbs may correspond to diabetic painful neuropathy (the most common type of neuropathy in the Western world). However, other types of pain, such as nociceptive/inflammatory pains (e.g., ulcers, osteoarthritis, and arterial disease), are frequent in patients with diabetes and may also involve the lower limbs (Figure 1.1; Table 1.1).

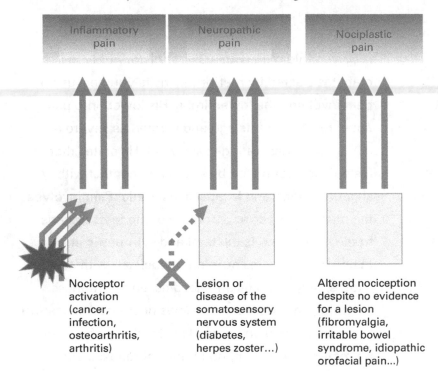

FIGURE 1.1 The three main chronic pain types. Nociceptive pain arises from actual or threatened damage to non-neural tissue and is due to the activation of nociceptors. This term is designed to contrast with neuropathic pain. The three arrows in the figure refer to increased nociceptor input arising from nociceptor activation (generally due to inflammation). Neuropathic pain is induced by a lesion or disease of the somatosensory nervous system. The hatched arrows suggest that neuropathic pain may arise despite partial to complete deafferentation (loss of afferent input). Common mechanisms include ectopic discharges generated in lesioned nerves or dorsal toot ganglia, central sensitization and dysfunction of modulatory controls. Nociplastic pain arises from altered nociception despite no clear evidence of actual or threatened tissue damage causing the activation of peripheral nociceptors or evidence for disease or lesion of the somatosensory system causing the pain. Of note, patients can have a combination of nociceptive, neuropathic, and nociplastic pain.

Source: Definitions from the International Association for the Study of Pain (https://www.iasp-pain.org/resources/terminology).

TABLE 1.1 Most Common Causes of Chronic Pains at the Lower Limbs in Patients with Diabetes

Nociceptive pains	Neuropathic pains
Osteoarthritis (knees, hips)[a]	Painful sensory or sensorimotor neuropathy
Peripheral arterial disease	Sciatica[a]
Ulcer, bedsores, infections	Femoral neuropathy
	Morton neuroma

[a]Not directly related to diabetes but frequent because of common risk factors (e.g., overweight).

To differentiate neuropathic pain in this diabetic patient from other types of pain, the characteristics of pain are essential. The patient describes his lower limb pain as "burning, electric shocks," worse by "contact with sheets," and associated with "tingling, pins and needles and numbness." These are typical neuropathic symptoms. Pain aggravated by contact with sheets suggests allodynia (pain induced by normally non-noxious stimuli), while tingling, pins and needles, and numbness, which are generally non-painful, correspond to paresthesia or dysesthesia (the latter refer to unpleasant sensations).

To assist in the diagnostic workup of neuropathic pain, you may employ an easy-to-use screening questionnaire. These questionnaires, which have been validated in multiple languages for routine use and are recommended by international scientific societies, all use common sensory terms and have up to 90% sensitivity and specificity to discriminate between neuropathic and non-neuropathic pains. They include the DN4 ("Douleur Neuropathique en 4 questions" also commonly called "Douleur Neuropathique 4 questionnaire"), the LANSS ("Leeds Assessment of Neuropathic Symptoms and Signs"), and PainDETECT. DN4 and LANSS include very simple bedside examination (using a brush and a pinprick for the area of pain), but self-reported forms (without examination) are also validated (DN4 interview and S-LANSS).

This patient score on his lower limb pain is 7/10 on the DN4 questionnaire (see Figure 1.2). This is higher than the cutoff score for detection of neuropathic pain (≥ 4/10) and suggests neuropathic pain (see Chapters 4 and 6 for examples of use of PainDETECT and LANSS).

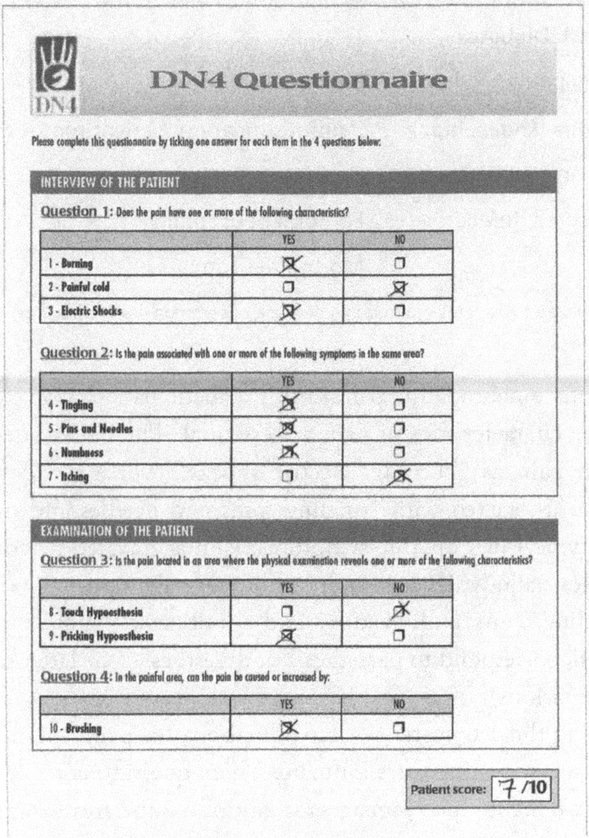

DN4 Questionnaire

Please complete this questionnaire by ticking one answer for each item in the 4 questions below:

INTERVIEW OF THE PATIENT

Question 1: Does the pain have one or more of the following characteristics?

	YES	NO
1 - Burning	☒	☐
2 - Painful cold	☐	☒
3 - Electric Shocks	☒	☐

Question 2: Is the pain associated with one or more of the following symptoms in the same area?

	YES	NO
4 - Tingling	☒	☐
5 - Pins and Needles	☒	☐
6 - Numbness	☒	☐
7 - Itching	☐	☒

EXAMINATION OF THE PATIENT

Question 3: Is the pain located in an area where the physical examination reveals one or more of the following characteristics?

	YES	NO
8 - Touch Hypoesthesia	☐	☒
9 - Pricking Hypoesthesia	☒	☐

Question 4: In the painful area, can the pain be caused or increased by:

	YES	NO
10 - Brushing	☒	☐

Patient score: 7 /10

FIGURE 1.2 Score obtained by the patient on the DN4 questionnaire. The score is 7 out of 10, which orients toward neuropathic pain (cutoff value for the detection of neuropathic pain is ≥ 4/10). The cutoff value for detection of neuropathic pain based on the DN4 interview (seven first items of the DN4 questionnaire) is ≥ 3/7.

To confirm the diagnosis, you may now (1) check for a link between pain onset and diabetes, (2) assess the exact pain area, and (3) complete the clinical examination.

1. The patient's pain appeared 18 months ago after his diabetes was diagnosed. Hence, there is a temporal link between the pain and diabetes.
2. Pain involves the plantar surface and dorsum of the feet, extends to the ankles, and is bilateral and symmetric. This corresponds to a

---

BOX 1.1　**Principles of Simple Bedside Sensory Examination in Patients Suspected of Neuropathic Pain**

1. Sensory examination should be conducted in the area of pain by comparison to the closest area of normal sensitivity. In patients with suspected sensory neuropathy, you may start from the most distal part of feet up to the knees to detect a change in sensitivity.
2. Thermoalgesic sensitivity (conveyed by small nociceptive fibers Aδ and C) may be tested by:
   - A pinprick (or disposable needle or 100-g monofilament) to detect decreased (or increased) pinprick sensation
   - Warm and cold tubes (or 20°C and 40°C thermorollers) to detect thermal deficits
3. Tactile/proprioceptive sensitivity (conveyed by large myelined Aβ fibers) may be tested by:
   - A brush to detect gross tactile deficit (crude touch) or abnormal pain sensation (allodynia)
   - A 10-g monofilament to detect fine tactile deficit
   - A 128-Hz tuning fork to detect vibration deficit
   - The search for impaired position sense of a body part to detect proprioceptive deficit (this may be completed by gait examination in search for proprioceptive ataxia)

"stocking" topography and is typical of the neuroanatomical area of sensory polyneuropathy.

3. The patient has decreased sensation to pinprick and pain induced by brushing (allodynia) in a stocking distribution in the painful area. This is compatible with a sensory neuropathy, but other sensory modalities may be assessed (Box 1.1 for principles of sensory examination). The lack of impairment of vibration sensation, motor deficit, or reflex abnormalities does not rule out the diagnosis of sensory neuropathy.

Of note, the fact that pain is severe and associated with insomnia has no diagnostic value.

Pain characteristics, medical history and context (diabetes), neuroanatomical area of pain, and findings of a sensory deficit in the painful area orient toward the diagnostic of probable painful diabetic neuropathy (according to an international diagnostic algorithm).

TABLE 1.2 Classification of Neuropathic Pains According to the International Association for the Study of Pain (2020)

Peripheral Neuropathic Pain	Central Neuropathic Pain
Trigeminal neuralgia[a]	Neuropathic pain associated with spinal cord injury
Neuropathic pain after peripheral nerve injury	Neuropathic pain associated with brain injury
Painful polyneuropathy	
Postherpetic neuralgia	Central post-stroke pain
Painful radiculopathy	Neuropathic pain associated with multiple sclerosis
Other peripheral neuropathic pain	Other central neuropathic pain

[a]Trigeminal neuralgia is classified as neuropathic pain but idiopathic trigeminal neuralgia has particular clinical characteristics and the sensory examination is generally normal (Chapter 19). Screening questionnaires are not suitable for trigeminal neuralgia.

There are many other causes of neuropathic pain (Table 1.2), and the diagnostic workup is generally similar for these pain conditions.

Complementary investigations may sometimes be necessary to confirm the diagnosis of the lesion responsible for the pain (this would fit the diagnosis of definite neuropathic pain). However, in this patient with typical clinical presentation, it is not mandatory to perform electromyography (EMG). Furthermore, EMG may be normal at early stages of diabetic neuropathies. Conversely, even if EMG shows a sensory neuropathy, this will not confirm neuropathic pain if pain has no neuropathic characteristics. Many patients with diabetes have subclinical neuropathy or painless neuropathy on EMG. Thus, EMG is confirmatory but should never replace clinical assessment.

KEY POINTS TO REMEMBER

· Neuropathic pain has particular clinical characteristics (e.g., burning, electric shocks, tingling, pins and needles, numbness, itch, and allodynia to touch) that differentiate it from nociceptive pains.

- Initial detection of neuropathic pain in routine may be aided by screening questionnaires such as the DN4, LANSS, or PainDETECT, which are mainly based on the characteristics of pain.
- To confirm the diagnosis of neuropathic pain, assessment of the clinical context and the area of pain, and sensory examination are mandatory.

Further Reading

Attal N, Bouhassira D, Baron R. Diagnosis and assessment of neuropathic pain through questionnaires. *Lancet Neurol.* 2018;17:456–466.

Attal N, Fermanian C, Fermanian J, et al. Neuropathic pain: Are there distinct subtypes depending on the aetiology or anatomical lesion? *Pain.* 2008;138:343–353.

Colloca L, Ludman T, Bouhassira D, et al. Neuropathic pain. *Nat Rev Dis Primers.* 2017;3:17002.

Finnerup NB, Haroutounian S, Kamerman P, et al. Neuropathic pain: An updated grading system for research and clinical practice. *Pain.* 2016;157:1599–1606.

Scholz J, Finnerup NB, Attal N, et al.; Classification Committee of the Neuropathic Pain Special Interest Group (NeuPSIG). The IASP classification of chronic pain for ICD-11: Chronic neuropathic pain. *Pain.* 2019;160:53–59.

Themistocleous AC, Ramirez JD, Shillo PR, et al. The Pain in Neuropathy Study (PiNS): A cross-sectional observational study determining the somatosensory phenotype of painful and painless diabetic neuropathy. *Pain.* 2016;157:1132–1145.

2 How to Implement First-Line Therapeutic Management

Nadine Attal and Didier Bouhassira

A 68-year-old overweight woman (BMI 31) has long-standing diabetic painful neuropathy. She reports chronic pain involving both legs (from the feet to mid thighs) and, to a lesser extent, the hands bilaterally. Pain is continuous, severe (numeric rating scale 7/10), mainly described as burning. She has used acetaminophen and ibuprofen without any efficacy and then tried paracetamol combined with codeine, but the latter was stopped because of constipation. She does not want any drug that might increase her weight or induce somnolence; she would like to still be able to read, travel, and look after her grandchildren.

What do you do now?

This woman suffers from painful diabetic neuropathy, a common cause of neuropathic pain. She has not responded to conventional analgesics. This is not surprising because conventional analgesics, including paracetamol, nonsteroidal anti-inflammatory drugs, and weak opioids, are poorly effective for painful diabetic neuropathy, due to the specific mechanisms of neuropathic pain. Hence, the World Health Organization's analgesic ladder is not adapted for neuropathic pain.

For this patient, based on international recommendations, you have the choice as first line in primary care between antidepressants and antiepileptics (Chapter 27). Antidepressants effective in painful diabetic neuropathy include tricyclic antidepressants (amitriptyline, imipramine, clomipramine, nortriptyline, and desipramine (10–150 mg per day, reduce doses in elderly patients) and drugs inhibiting the reuptake of serotonin and noradrenalin, particularly duloxetine (60–120 mg once daily), whereas other antidepressants are poorly effective. Antiepileptics with best evidence for efficacy are gabapentin (900–3600 mg per day) and pregabalin (150–600 mg per day) (Table 2.1). Gapabentin enacarbil, a prodrug of gabapentin, has been found effective in postherpetic neuralgia.

This woman is afraid of being somnolent and gaining weight. Hence, tricyclic agents, pregabalin, or gabapentin is not ideal due to the risk of somnolence and increased weight (Table 2.1). We advise you to consider oral duloxetine (U.S. Food and Drug Administration [FDA] approved for diabetic painful neuropathy) with has a different side effect profile (Table 2.1). You may start with 30 mg daily during meals (to limitate the risk of nausea) for 7 days and then titrate up to 60 mg daily. In this woman, the drug had acceptable efficacy (50%) for her burning pain at 60 mg per day and was well tolerated except for mild initial nausea.

The following is general guidance regarding therapeutic management of neuropathic pain including painful diabetic neuropathy, based on evidence or expert consensus (Figure 2.1):

- Neuropathic pain generally does not respond to conventional analgesics.
- The treatment of neuropathic pain is minimally dependent on the etiology of pain because the mechanisms of pain are common to multiple etiologies. Recommendations suitable for this woman

TABLE 2.1 **Drugs Recommended as First Line for Neuropathic Pain in Adults in Primary Care**

Drug, Dosages, and Official Approval for Use in Analgesia	Mechanisms of Action	Adverse Effects	Main Precautions for Use and Contraindications
Tricyclic Antidepressants			
Amitriptyline, clomipramine, imipramine, nortriptyline, desipramine 10–150 mg once daily or in 2 divided doses (reduce doses in elderly) FDA: no approval in analgesia Europe: approved in select countries for neuropathic pain	Inhibits reuptake of monoamines; may also act as sodium channel blockers; anticholinergic effects	Somnolence, confusion, sweating, dry mouth, dysuria, constipation, weight gain, sexual effects, hyponatremia, increased liver enzyme, seizures. Nortriptyline and desipramine less somnolence/confusion	Cardiac disease (recent myocardial infarction and QT prolongation) (ECG), narrow angle glaucoma, prostatic adenoma, seizures. Avoid tertiary amines (amitriptyline, clomipramine, imipramine) at doses ≥75 mg/day after age 65 years. ECG recommended to assess QT interval FDA blackbox (suicide risk)
Serotonin–Norepinephrine Reuptake Inhibitors			
Duloxetine 60–120 mg once daily or in 2 divided doses FDA: DPN and chronic musculoskeletal pain EMA: DPN	Inhibits reuptake of serotonin and norepinephrine	Nausea, abdominal pain, constipation, insomnia, sexual effects, increased liver enzymes, hyponatrema	Severe hepatic disorder, unstable hypertension Concomitant use of tramadol FDA blackbox (suicide risk)

(continued)

TABLE 2.1 **Continued**

Drug, Dosages, and Official Approval for Use in Analgesia	**Mechanisms of Action**	**Adverse Effects**	**Main Precautions for Use and Contraindications**
Antiepileptics			
Gabapentin 1200–3600 mg per day in 3 divided doses FDA: DPN/PHN EMA: peripheral NP Gabapentin enacarbil (extended release tablets) 1200 mg per day (once daily) FDA: PHN Pregabalin 150–600 mg per day in 2 or 3 divided doses FDA: DPN/PHN/spinal cord injury pain EMA: peripheral/central NP	Acts on α₂δ subunit of voltage-gated calcium channels	Somnolence, dizziness, peripheral edema, weight gain. Abuse reported (mainly pregabalin)	Reduce dose in renal insufficiency Contraindicated in severe renal insufficiency Abuse potential Risk of respiratory depression in combination with high doses of opioids Scheduled drugs in the United Kingdom

DPN, diabetic painful neuropathy; ECG, electrocardiogram; EMA, European Medicines Agency; NP, neuropathic pain; PHN, postherpetic neuralgia.

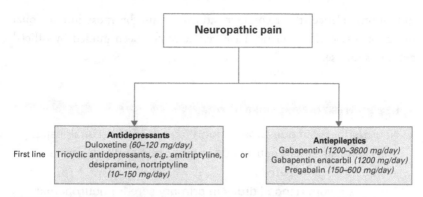

FIGURE 2.1 Therapeutic algorithm for first-line pharmacotherapy of neuropathic pain in primary care. Duloxetine, pregabalin, and gabapentin are FDA approved for use in at least one neuropathic pain indication (see Table 2.1).

Modified from Finnerup et al. (2015) and Moisset et al. (2020).

with diabetic painful neuropathy are generally applicable to other neuropathic pain conditions (see Chapter 1) with the exception of trigeminal neuralgia.

- All oral drug therapies for neuropathic pain should be increased gradually up to efficacy or side effects (individual titration).
- Drug treatments should be proposed as monotherapy and then first-line drugs may be combined in case of limited efficacy (e.g., pregagalin with duloxetine or tricyclic antidepressants; gabapentin with duloxetine or tricyclic antidepressants), but it is not recommended to combine drugs from the same class (e.g., two antidepressants).
- In case of efficacy, you should continue the treatment for at least 6 months and then taper off therapy.
- You should never stop oral drug treatments abruptly because of the risk of withdrawal syndrome.

Unfortunately, not all drugs recommended for neuropathic pain have specific approvals for use, and approvals also vary according to countries or continents (Table 2.1). For example, FDA approvals are limited to three etiologies of neuropathic pain in adults—diabetic painful neuropathies, postherpetic neuralgia, and spinal cord injury pain—even though neuropathic pain encompasses a much larger variety of etiologies (see Chapter 1) and these drugs have been shown to be effective in other neuropathic pain indications. Hence, the recommendations for use by most international or national scientific societies have generally not been guided by official approvals for use.

KEY POINTS TO REMEMBER

- Neuropathic pain does not respond to conventional analgesics.
- The management of neuropathic pain is minimally dependent on the etiology of pain.
- First-line recommended drugs in primary care for neuropathic pain include antidepressants (duloxetine, and tricyclic antidepressants such as amitriptyline) and gabapentinoids (gabapentin or pregabalin).
- Oral drugs should be proposed as monotherapy first under the principle of individual titration (increase the doses up to side effects or efficacy).
- Oral drugs should not be discontinued abruptly but tapered off slowly after at least 6 months in case of efficacy.

Further Reading

Attal N, Bouhassira D. Advances in the treatment of neuropathic pain. *Curr Opin Neurol.* 2021;34(5):631–637.

Attal N, Fermanian C, Fermanian J, et al. Neuropathic pain: Are there distinct subtypes depending on the aetiology or anatomical lesion? *Pain.* 2008;138(2):343–353.

Colloca L, Ludman T, Bouhassira D, et al. Neuropathic pain. *Nat Rev Dis Primers.* 2017;3:17002.

Finnerup NB, Attal N, Haroutounian S, et al. Pharmacotherapy for neuropathic pain in adults: A systematic review and meta-analysis. *Lancet Neurol.* 2015;14(2):162–173.

Moisset X, Bouhassira D, Avez Couturier J, et al. Pharmacological and non-pharmacological treatments for neuropathic pain: Systematic review and French recommendations. *Rev Neurol.* 2020;176(5):325–352.

3 Itch and Herpes Zoster

Michael C. Rowbotham

An 85-year-old woman experienced unilateral intense
eye and facial pain a few days after Christmas.
Her vision began to blur and severe itching on the
forehead was followed 2 days later by a vesicular
rash. Her physician diagnosed herpes zoster,
started her on oral acyclovir, and referred her to an
ophthalmologist. Examination found keratitis but
intact vision. She received steroid eyedrops and
oral hydrocodone/acetaminophen combination (up
to 30 mg per day). By 3 months, the rash was gone
and her vision had cleared but she still suffered
severe pain and itch despite her treatment. . . . She
now describes intractable itching throughout the
hyperpigmented area where she had the rash and a
sensation of sand in her eyes, improved by wearing
sunglasses. She is extremely sensitive to touch and
wind. Her pain is described as constant burning with
severe lancinating pain (10 times a day). Otherwise,
she has no sad mood and states that yoga helps her
cope with her pain.

What do you do now?

This elderly woman suffers from persistent neuropathic pain and itch 3 months after acute ophthalmic zoster, despite healing of her skin lesions in the area of her acute herpes zoster rash (the face). She meets criteria for postherpetic neuralgia (PHN). She is experiencing burning pain, lancinating pains, evoked pain (allodynia) to tactile stimulation (touch and wind), severe itch, and eye pain. Neuropathic itch (which is a symptom of neuropathic pain, see Chapter 1) is particularly frequent in PHN, may even be worse than spontaneous pain, and may share mechanisms with pain. Brush evoked pain or pain evoked by wind (mechanical allodynia) is also frequent and may be the most distressing symptom. Lancinating pains (often described as electric shocks) are the most likely to resolve spontaneously, whereas other pain symptoms and sensory deficit may persist for months, particularly because of her older age (the strongest risk factor for PHN), severity of her acute infection (another major risk factor for PHN), and pain location (ophthalmic area) (Figure 3.1).

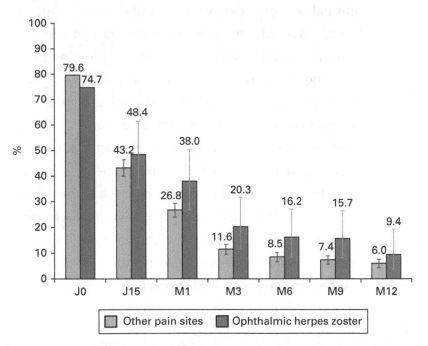

FIGURE 3.1 Prevalence of pain after ophtalmic herpes zoster compared to other pain sites.

Adapted and modified from Bouhassira et al. (2012).

This woman also reports that wearing sunglasses improves her sensation of sand in her eyes. Nonmedicated protective ointments may indeed have a small therapeutic role, as do sunglasses, headscarves, and hats (that do not put pressure on forehead skin). Otherwise, this woman does not suffer from major depression or social isolation, which might have aggravated her pain.

You should first ask this woman if she has been back to see the ophthalmologist. Enduring anterior and even posterior eye damage is indeed not uncommon after herpes zoster. Chronic keratitis must be searched for. This woman had seen an ophthalmologist and had no keratitis or reduced visual acuity.

How do you manage this woman's neuropathic pain and itch? She has only received low-dose opioids. Weak opioids are generally ineffective for neuropathic pain and itch, but they may have a place for acute herpes zoster when pain is both inflammatory and neuropathic (and were probably initially helpful). A conversion to a long-acting opioid might be possible but certainly not as the first step. You should try a gabapentinoid, pregabalin, or gabapentin (U.S. Food and Drug Administration [FDA] and European Medicines Agency [EMA] approval for use [Chapter 2]; patients may respond differently to each, and either one can be tried first), an antidepressant (tricyclic antidepressants or duloxetine; no FDA approval in PHN), or lidocaine 5% plasters (FDA approved for PHN, generally recommended as second line, first line for frail and elderly patients).

After checking for creatinine clearance (45 μmol/l), this woman was first treated by low-dose gabapentin (100 mg) titrated upward by steps of 100 mg every 7 days up to 600 mg TID. She reported moderate analgesic efficacy (30%) and severe somnolence and dizziness, which are usual side effects of the drug, and preferred to stop the treatment. Pregabalin was not proposed because she had not tolerated gabapentin (both drugs have similar side effect profile), and tricyclic antidepressants were not advised because of significant risk at her age (falls and cardiotoxicity), although very low dosages in the evening, such as 10 mg per day, might have been at tempted. Lidocaine plasters were then proposed (one plaster for 12 consecutive hours) because her pain area was limited, although they are difficult to use on the face and should not be used for eye or scalp pain (main side effects are local allergy). Here, they were well tolerated and had acceptable efficacy on facial pain and itch (40%). Of note, other topical therapies have a limited role for trigeminal PHN. Thus, capsaicin (low-concentration creams or high-concentration patches) is not recommended for the face (capsaicin that gets into the conjunctiva produces intense pain) but recommended as second line for PHN affecting other body areas, such as the thoracic area (FDA and EMA approval in this indication). Anti-itch topicals that do not contain local anesthetics generally fail due to the neuropathic nature of the PHN itch.

Ophthalmic zoster makes up approximately 15–20% of all acute herpes zoster cases and is more likely to progress to PHN compared to acute herpes zoster in other body locations (the latter concern mainly the thorax, then lumbar and cervical areas, and seldom the genitals; disseminated rash is exceptional, except in immunocompromised patients) (Figure 3.1). Anyone who has had natural infection with varicella zoster virus (VZV) or had varicella vaccination can develop herpes zoster, but children who get the varicella vaccine (available in the United States) have a lower risk of herpes zoster. Of note, 99.5% of people born before 1980 in the United States have been infected with wild-type VZV. As a result, almost all older adults in the United States are at risk for herpes zoster. The intense suffering experienced by patients with trigeminal PHN emphasizes the importance of ensuring everyone aged 50 years or older receives the two-dose Shingrix recombinant DNA vaccine (97% effective in preventing herpes zoster). With the Zostavax vaccine, which was approximately 70% effective, cases of zoster were milder and much less likely to result in PHN. Although an episode of shingles boosts immunity and reduces the likelihood of another bout of zoster, current recommendations are that the woman receives the two-dose Shingrix vaccine once she is no longer acutely ill. Preventing shingles prevents PHN.

KEY POINTS TO REMEMBER

- The best treatment for PHN is prevention of shingles. All eligible persons should be vaccinated. Reported efficacy for both zoster and PHN is greater than 90% for the Shingrix (lower for Zostavax).

- All patients with trigeminal zoster need an evaluation and careful follow-up by an ophthalmologist.
- Topical therapies including 5% lidocaine plasters are a good option for postherpetic neuralgia but have a more limited role for trigeminal PHN than thoracic PHN.
- Gabapentinoids are approved for trigeminal PHN, but relief may be incomplete.
- Tricyclic antidepressants carry the greatest risks but are effective. Serotonin–norepinephrine reuptake inhibitor antidepressants such as duloxetine are not necessarily better tolerated but safer.
- Supportive and nonmedication therapies have a major role in management of trigeminal PHN.
- Invasive or destructive therapies have little or no role.

Further Reading

Finnerup NB, Attal N, Haroutounian S, et al. Pharmacotherapy for neuropathic pain in adults: A systematic review and meta-analysis. *Lancet Neurol.* 2015;14(2):162–173.

Mallick-Searle T, Snodgrass B, Brant J. Postherpetic neuralgia: Epidemiology, pathophysiology, and pain management pharmacology. *J Multidiscip Healthc.* 2016;9:447–454. https://doi.org/10.2147/JMDH.S106340

Oaklander AL, Cohen SP, Raju, SVY. Intractable postherpetic itch and cutaneous deafferentation after facial shingles, *Pain.* 2002; 96(1):9–12.

Rowbotham MC, Fields HL. Post-herpetic neuralgia: The relation of pain complaint, sensory disturbance, and skin temperature. *Pain.* 1989;39:129–144.

Rowbotham MC, Harden N, Stacey B, Bernstein P, Magnus-Miller L. Gabapentin for the treatment of postherpetic neuralgia. *JAMA.* 1998;280:1837–1842.

Sugar O, Bucy PC. Postherpetic trigeminal neuralgia. *Arch Neurol Psychiatry.* 1951;65:131–145.

Vrcek I, Choudhury E, Durairaj V. Herpes zoster ophthalmicus: A review for the internist. *Am J Med.* 2017;130:21–26. http://dx.doi.org/10.1016/j.amj med.2016.08.039

4 Chronic Low Back and Leg Pain

Nadine Attal and Didier Bouhassira

A 48-year-old woman was operated for L4–L5 left discal herniation 2 years ago because of acute sciatica and paresis of the foot. Her past history includes vein thrombosis treated with warfarin and narrow-angle glaucoma. Despite surgery, she suffers from continuous moderate low back pain described as heavy and cramping, and severe continuous pain at the leg (posterior and lateral aspects of the thigh and leg up to the dorsum of the foot), described as burning, electric shocks, and associated with tingling. She walks slowly because she is afraid that any movement might aggravate her pain. Sensory examination discloses reduced pinprick sensation in the leg and evoked pain to brush at the dorsum of the foot. There is no motor deficit, reflex abnormalities, or Lasègue's sign. Lumbar magnetic resonance imaging (MRI) does not show new discal herniation. She has not responded to acetaminophen, nonsteroidal anti-inflammatory drugs (NSAIDs), and epidural corticosteroids and does not tolerate weak opioids.

What do you do now?

This woman has chronic low back pain and lower limb pain despite surgery. Her low back pain is described as heavy, cramping, and not associated with sensory deficit, whereas her leg pain is described as burning, electric shocks, sensitive to touch, and associated with tingling, which suggests neuropathic characteristics. This may be confirmed by a screening questionnaire such as DN4 or PainDETECT (see Chapter 1). Here, the score of PainDETECT is 6 for the lower back and 25 for the leg ($\geq$ 19, cutoff score for likely neuropathic pain), suggesting that only her lower limb pain is neuropathic (Figure 4.1).

This woman's lower limb pain extends below the knee up to the foot in the posterior and lateral aspects of the thigh and leg, which corresponds to the L5 left territory and suggests radicular pain. This is confirmed by sensory examination of the leg disclosing reduced sensation to pinprick in the L5 territory and pain evoked by light brush (allodynia) at the dorsum at the foot.

Based on clinical context (surgery), pain location, and pain characteristics and examination, the best diagnosis is chronic painful radiculopathy (or failed back surgery syndrome because this woman was operated on) (Table 4.1). The absence of Lasègue's sign does not rule out radiculopathy because this sign indicates radicular compression, and root compression was removed by spinal surgery. The mechanisms of her radicular pain probably involve adhesions, ischemia, or arachnoiditis. MRI or computed tomography scan is required to rule out potential other causes for pain, in case of motor deficit. Electromyography (EMG) is not mandatory because she has typical radicular pain.

How do you manage this woman's pain? You should advise her to start physical reconditioning because deconditioning may have contributed to her residual low back pain. You may ask for psychological advice and recommend cognitive–behavioral therapy because she is afraid of movement. Transcutaneous electrical nerve stimulation may be proposed for her leg pain (US. Food and Drug Administration [FDA] approved) (see Chapter 33). First-line drugs include gabapentin, pregabalin, tricyclic antidepressants (amitriptyline), or duloxetine (no FDA approval in this indication; see Chapter 2 for official approvals for use). You should not propose opioids as first line, and conventional analgesics and NSAIDs are generally ineffective for chronic radicular pain (they may be proposed for acute pain). The utility of lumbar

(a)

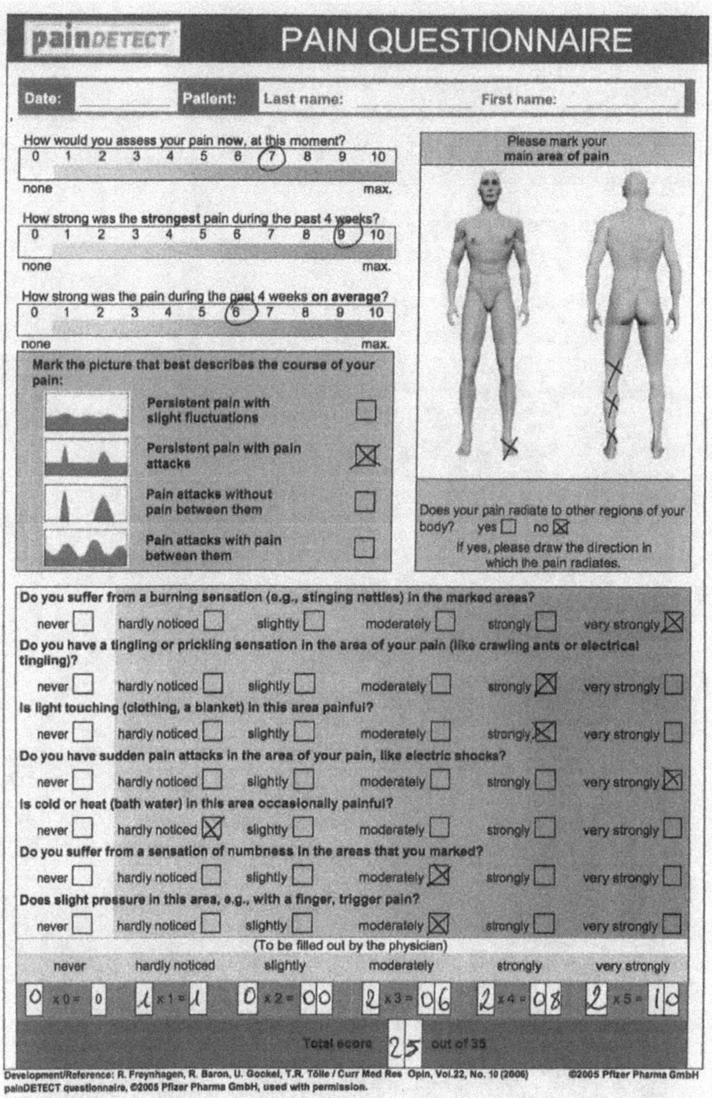

FIGURE 4.1 Results of the PainDETECT screening questionnaire (see Chapter 1) at the leg (A) and at the lower back (B) in this patient. Neuropathic pain is likely for a cutoff value ≥ 19 on this questionnaire. The total score is 6 for the lower back and 25 for the leg, suggesting that only the lower limb pain is neuropathic.

(b)

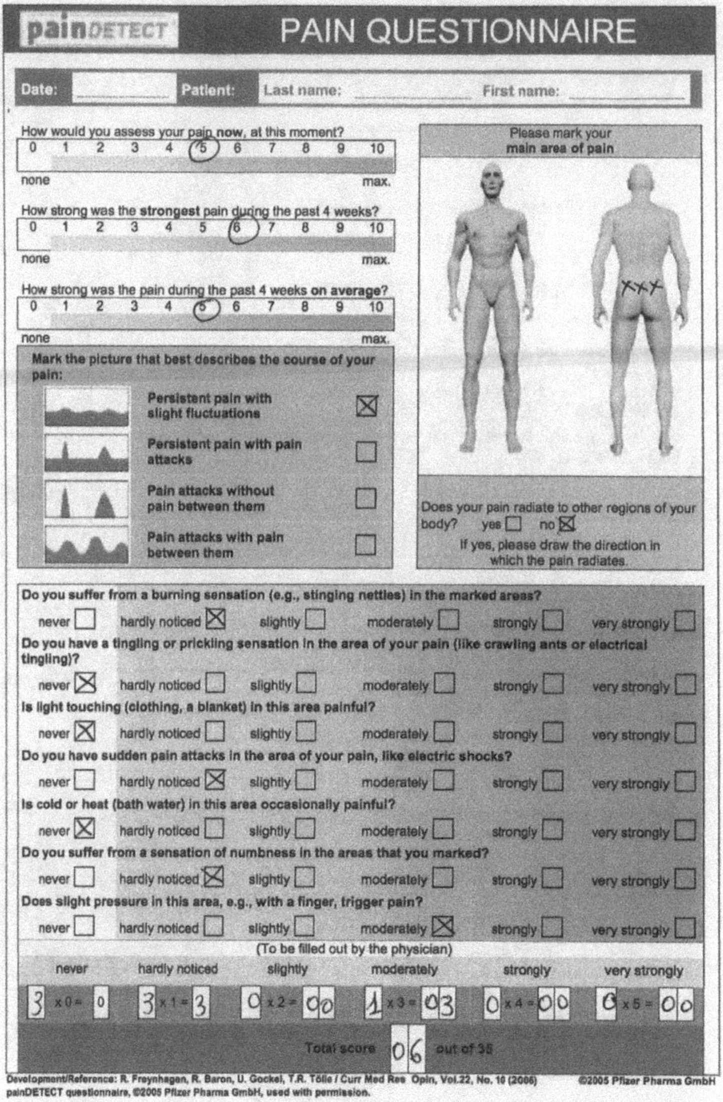

painDETECT   PAIN QUESTIONNAIRE

Date: Patient: Last name: First name:

How would you assess your pain now, at this moment?

| 0 | 1 | 2 | 3 | 4 | (5) | 6 | 7 | 8 | 9 | 10 |

none   max.

How strong was the **strongest** pain during the past 4 weeks?

| 0 | 1 | 2 | 3 | 4 | 5 | (6) | 7 | 8 | 9 | 10 |

none   max.

How strong was the pain during the past 4 weeks **on average**?

| 0 | 1 | 2 | 3 | 4 | (5) | 6 | 7 | 8 | 9 | 10 |

none   max.

Please mark your main area of pain

Mark the picture that best describes the course of your pain:

- Persistent pain with slight fluctuations ☒
- Persistent pain with pain attacks ☐
- Pain attacks without pain between them ☐
- Pain attacks with pain between them ☐

Does your pain radiate to other regions of your body? yes ☐ no ☒

If yes, please draw the direction in which the pain radiates.

Do you suffer from a burning sensation (e.g., stinging nettles) in the marked areas?

never ☐   hardly noticed ☒   slightly ☐   moderately ☐   strongly ☐   very strongly ☐

Do you have a tingling or prickling sensation in the area of your pain (like crawling ants or electrical tingling)?

never ☒   hardly noticed ☐   slightly ☐   moderately ☐   strongly ☐   very strongly ☐

Is light touching (clothing, a blanket) in this area painful?

never ☒   hardly noticed ☐   slightly ☐   moderately ☐   strongly ☐   very strongly ☐

Do you have sudden pain attacks in the area of your pain, like electric shocks?

never ☐   hardly noticed ☒   slightly ☐   moderately ☐   strongly ☐   very strongly ☐

Is cold or heat (bath water) in this area occasionally painful?

never ☒   hardly noticed ☐   slightly ☐   moderately ☐   strongly ☐   very strongly ☐

Do you suffer from a sensation of numbness in the areas that you marked?

never ☐   hardly noticed ☒   slightly ☐   moderately ☐   strongly ☐   very strongly ☐

Does slight pressure in this area, e.g., with a finger, trigger pain?

never ☐   hardly noticed ☐   slightly ☐   moderately ☒   strongly ☐   very strongly ☐

(To be filled out by the physician)

never	hardly noticed	slightly	moderately	strongly	very strongly
3 x 0 = 0	3 x 1 = 3	0 x 2 = 00	1 x 3 = 03	0 x 4 = 00	0 x 5 = 00

Total score   06   out of 35

Development/Reference: R. Freynhagen, R. Baron, U. Gockel, T.R. Tölle / Curr Med Res Opin, Vol.22, No. 10 (2006)   ©2005 Pfizer Pharma GmbH
painDETECT questionnaire, ©2005 Pfizer Pharma GmbH, used with permission.

FIGURE 4.1 Continued

TABLE 4.1   Main Characteristics of Chronic Radicular Pain (i.e., Sciatica, Femoral Neuralgia, and Cervicobrachial Neuralgia)

Pain characteristics	Neuropathic characteristics: burning, cold, electric shocks, tingling, pins and needles, pricking, numbness, itchy, sensitive to touch.
Pain distribution	Neuroanatomical area corresponding to the distribution of a radicular nerve but in very chronic cases may expand outside a neuroanatomical distribution.
Clinical examination	Sensory deficit in the painful area: generally pinprick, hot or cold but may be normal. Allodynia to brush is also common. Motor deficits and fine tactile or vibration deficits are more uncommon. Tendon reflexes may be normal or impaired if the lesion involves S1 impairment at the lower limbs or C6–C8 at the upper limbs.
EMG	May show radiculopathy or be normal if the lesion spares large myelinated fibers. EMG is not mandatory in the case of typical clinical presentation.

epidural steroid injections is controversial in chronic radicular pain. Although effective in certain patient populations, these treatments have been associated with serious complications, including paralysis and death. In 2014, the FDA issued a safety warning on the risk of injecting corticosteroids into the epidural space, and the risk is increased after spinal surgery.

An adequate first-line treatment option in this woman is gabapentin because it has no drug–drug interaction and may improve her sleep and generalized anxiety. Duloxetine is not recommended because it would interact with warfarin, and tricyclic antidepressants are contraindicated because of her narrow-angle glaucoma. With lack of renal insufficiency, you should initiate gabapentin at 300 mg daily in the evening (100 mg in case of moderate renal insufficiency or patient age older than 75 years) and then increase by increments of 300 mg every 4–7 days (depending on efficacy and side effects) for up to 1200 mg to a maximum of 3600 mg per day (usual average dosage is 1800 mg per day). Main side effects include dizziness, somnolence, weight gain, and peripheral edema. You may also use pregabalin (starting with 75 mg in the evening—less in case of renal impairment—and then increasing by increments of 75 mg every 4–7 days up to 150–600 mg per day). These drugs should not be combined together because they have the same mechanisms of action.

This woman received gabapentin up to 1200 mg per day. She reports acceptable efficacy (50%) for her leg pain, particularly on her electric shocks. Her back pain persists but is slowly improving with balneotherapy. She continues to have moderate burning pain in the leg, but her residual pain is judged tolerable. You may continue gabapentin for at least 6 months and then taper off therapy progressively if the pain is minimal.

Low back pain is the main cause of burden of illness with a 1-month prevalence of 24%. It most commonly affects middle-aged to older women. In the United States, costs associated with the management of patients with low back pain are estimated to exceed $100 billion annually. Radicular pain is the most common cause of neuropathic pain in the general population, according to epidemiological studies. The prevalence of neuropathic pain ranges between 16% and 55% in patients with chronic low back pain. Radicular pain is most commonly associated with discal herniation and spinal stenosis generally at the L4–L5 level, particularly after age 60 years. The latter is an anatomically progressive condition resulting from facet joint hypertrophy, congenitally short pedicles, and spondylolisthesis. However, the presence of a herniated disc does not always result in pain, and most regress spontaneously within 2 years. Spinal stenosis is also commonly found in asymptomatic subjects. This means that surgery should probably not be undertaken because of pain but, rather, because of motor or sphincter deficits (the latter suggesting cauda equina syndrome in the case of lumbosacral disc herniation).

KEY POINTS TO REMEMBER

· Chronic low back pain and leg pain involve nociceptive and neuropathic mechanisms.
· Failed back surgery syndrome corresponds to persisting back and leg pain despite surgery.

- Screening instruments such as DN4 and PainDETECT may help differentiate neuropathic and nociceptive low back and leg pain with high specificity and sensitivity.
- Therapeutic management of chronic failed back surgery syndrome should be guided by pain mechanisms. For neuropathic (radicular) pain, recommendations should follow general guidelines for peripheral neuropathic pain and should include as first line drugs such as pregabalin, gabapentin, amitriptyline, or duloxetine; opioids should not be prescribed as first line.

Further Reading

Attal N, Perrot S, Fermanian J, Bouhassira D. The neuropathic components of chronic low back pain: A prospective multicenter study using the DN4 Questionnaire. *J Pain.* 2011;12(10):1080–1087.

Cohen SP, Greuber E, Vought K, Lissin D. Safety of epidural steroid injections for lumbosacral radicular pain: Unmet medical need. *Clin J Pain.* 2021;37(9):707–717.

Knezevic NN, Candido KD, Vlaeyen JWS, Van Zundert J, Cohen SP. Low back pain. *Lancet.* 2021;398(10294):78–92.

Mathieson S, Maher CG, McLachlan AJ, et al. Trial of pregabalin for acute and chronic sciatica. *N Engl J Med.* 2017;376(12):1111–1120.

Oliveira CB, Maher CG, Ferreira ML, et al. Epidural corticosteroid injections for lumbosacral radicular pain. *Cochrane Database Syst Rev.* 2020;4(4):CD013577.

Robertson K, Marshman LAG, Plummer D, Downs E. Effect of gabapentin vs. pregabalin on pain intensity in adults with chronic sciatica: A randomized clinical trial. *JAMA Neurol.* 2019;76(1):28–34.

5 Painful Legs and Diabetes (1)

Nadine Attal and Didier Bouhassira

A 48-year-old man responsible for a wine business has type II diabetes (within 10 years) with poor diabetic control. His past history includes myocardial infarction and smoking (stopped after his infarction). He reports drinking several glasses of wine per day for business lunches. His pain started 4 years ago. It is bilateral and symmetrical at both feet, enhanced at night and by walking, described as cold/ice, itch, pins and needles, and pricking. At examination he is 178 cm tall and weighs 128 kg (body mass index >40). He states that he gained 40 pounds because of gabapentin. Examination shows sensory deficit to brush and pinprick, reduced vibration sense at the feet, and absent ankle reflexes. Peripheral pulses are present and there are no skin abnormalities. Electromyography (EMG) shows sensory neuropathy. Blood tests show elevated increased γ-glutamyl transferase, and macrocytosis. He would like to get rid of his pain completely.

What do you do now?

This man suffers from neuropathic pain at the legs. Pain is bilateral and symmetrical at both feet, and it is situated in an area of sensory deficit. EMG shows sensory neuropathy. He has no other apparent reasons to account for his pain, such as ulcerations or trophic changes at the feet or arteriopathy, and his blood tests show biological counterparts of his alcoholic use. The diagnosis is compatible with diabetic and/or alcoholic painful neuropathy (see Table 5.1 for other causes of neuropathic pain in diabetic patients).

You should first ask this patient to optimize his glycemic control, lose weight, and abstain from alcohol, but this is probably easier said than done. Psychoeducation is essential. This man has to accept that it will take months or even years before he sees an (potential) impact of reducing his alcohol consumption and optimizing glycemic control on his neuropathy. He also has to understand that no treatment will allow him to get totally rid of his pain but that the goal of therapy is to help him reduce his pain (by 30–50% generally). Before he loses weight and starts reducing his alcohol consumption, he may start a symptomatic treatment. Thiamine (B$_1$ vitamin) or benfotiamine, a synthetic prodrug of thiamine, might be relevant. Other pathogenic-derived pharmacotherapy, such as aldose reductase inhibitors or α-lipoic acid, may be tried depending on their availability, but their long-term efficacy has yet to be confirmed.

For his pain, the patient has tried FDA-approved gabapentin, which caused weight gain and peripheral edema. Other first-line recommended drug treatments for diabetic painful neuropathies include tricyclic antidepressants (amitriptyline, nortriptyline, or desipramine 10–150 mg per day), FDA-approved duloxetine (60–120 mg per day), or FDA-approved pregabalin (150–600 mg per day) (see Chapter 2). However, tricyclic antidepressants and pregabalin may also cause increased weight (and pregabalin has the same risk of peripheral edema as gabapentin), and duloxetine may induce liver injury particularly in patients with preexisting liver disease or chronic alcohol use. Hence, because the patient's pain is limited to the feet, we advise you to consider either transcutaneous electrical nerve stimulation (if he haves access to it) (see Chapter 33) or off-label 5% lidocaine plasters (FDA and EMA approved in postherpetic neuralgia) which are generally recommended as second line for patients with peripheral neuropathic pain and limited pain area (Table 5.2; Figure 5.1).

TABLE 5.1　Main Types of Neuropathic Pain in Patients with Diabetes and Their Description

Neuropathy Types	Description
Chronic painful distal sensorimotor polyneuropathy (the most common)	Symmetrical, length-dependent sensorimotor polyneuropathy, beginning in both toes and then feet and legs in a "stocking distribution." Subsequently, the upper limbs can be affected. Motor manifestations may follow sensory loss. Concerns one-third of patients (13–34% in developed countries, higher in type II diabetes). Potential role of hyperglycemia, dyslipidemia, and microvascular disease; ectopic discharges and central sensitization relevant mechanisms for pain. Main risk factors (for painful neuropathy), including duration of diabetes, metabolic syndrome, and female sex. Diagnosis mainly clinical based on symptoms (e.g., quality and area of pain) and signs (sensory examination using light touch, pinprick, temperature, vibration; motor function; tendon reflexes). Questionnaires such as the Michigan Neuropathy Screening Instrument may confirm diabetic neuropathy.
Acute painful distal sensory polyneuropathies	In the context of poor diabetic control (generally associated with weight loss) or after rapid improvements in glucose control. Typical presentation: acute "stocking and glove" pain distribution. Management should focus on relieving pain and maintenance of optimal glycemic control.
Focal or multifocal neuropathies	Caused by nerve compression or microvasculitis. May be difficult to distinguish from entrapment neuropathies; their diagnosis generally needs nerve conduction studies.
Mononeuropathy and mononeuritis multiplex	Cranial nerve palsies (e.g., third cranial nerve) are the most common and may be painful.

(*continued*)

TABLE 5.1 **Continued**

Neuropathy Types	Description
Radiculoplexopathy	Mostly lumbosacral radiculoplexopathy. Typical presentation: subacute unilateral lower limb neuropathy associated with weight loss and proximal muscle weakness or pain in a radicular distribution.
Entrapment neuropathies	Involve the median, ulnar, and peroneal nerves. Unilateral pain and paresthesia (e.g., tingling) affecting the corresponding dermatomas, often worse at night and triggered by maneuvers such as Tinel at the wrist. Diagnosis requires nerve conduction studies. Intermetatarsal neuroma or Morton's neuroma affects most commonly the third or fourth intermetatarsal space and is characterized by pain at walking and evoked by pressure of the third or fourth intermetatarsal space. Diagnosis generally requires tomography or magnetic resonance imaging of the foot.

Adapted and modified from Sloan et al. (2021).

This patient received lidocaine plasters (one patch per foot for 12 consecutive hours), but thought they were not practical during daytime and insufficient at night. He was then referred to a pain specialist, who proposed capsaicin high-concentration (8%) patches (FDA approved for diabetic painful neuropathies) (Table 5.2; Figure 5.1). After two repeated administrations every 3 months (one plaster and half per foot during 30 minutes), he reports substantial pain relief and continues to use this drug treatment regularly (every 3 months). He states that he is not depressed and does not need a psychologist, but he agrees to see a diabetologist. He also states that he is able to reduce alcohol without help from specialists. You have to monitor him carefully over time to see how he is able to cope with his disease and his alcohol use.

Although tramadol (sustained release tramadol should be preferred to immediate release tramadol) is also generally recommended as second line for neuropathic pain (Table 5.2; Fig. 5.1), you should avoid opioids in this patient with chronic alcoholic use. In case of therapeutic failure, you may

TABLE 5.2 Drugs generally Recommended as Second Line for Neuropathic Pain in Adults[a]

Drug, Dosages, and Official Approval for Use in Analgesia	Mechanism of Action	Adverse Effects	Main Precautions for Use and Contraindications
Local anaesthetics (for peripheral neuopathic pain only)			
5 % lidocaine plasters 1 to 3 plasters as per the pain area every day during up to 12 hours FDA and EMA : postherpetic neuralgia	Blockade of sodium channels	Irritation, erythema, cutaneous allergy	Difficult to use on the face Avoid in patients with skin lesion, injection, or irritation
Capsaicin (for peripheral neuropathic pain only, specialist use)			
Capsaicin high-concentration patches (8%) 1–4 (as per the pain area) every 2 or 3 months FDA: diabetic painful neuropathy of the feet/postherpetic neuralgia EMA: peripheral neuropathic pain	Transient receptor potential vanilloid 1 agonist; initial burning pain and edema (activation of C nociceptors), then nociceptor defunctionalization	Pain, erythema, itch, increased blood pressure (rare) during or after application (induced pain)	Difficult to use on the face. Avoid in patients with skin lesion, infection, or irritation
Opioids			
Tramadol (sustained-release) 200–400 mg per day FDA/EMA: moderate/severe pain	Mu receptor agonist and monoamine reuptake inhibition	Nausea, vomiting, constipation, dizziness, somnolence, abuse, seizures	History of substance abuse, suicide risk, use of antidepressants (particularly high dosages), patients aged ≥75 years (confusion), unstable seizures

[a]See Chapter 2 for first-line drugs.
EMA, European Medicines Agency.

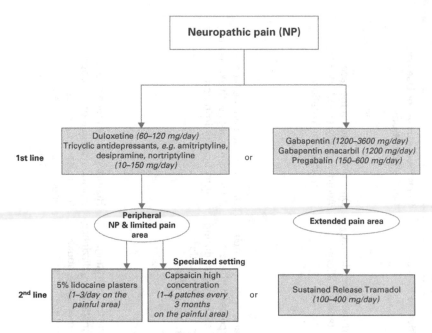

FIGURE 5.1 Therapeutic algorithm for first- and second-line pharmacotherapy of neuropathic pain in primary and secondary care. Second-line drugs include topical agents (e.g., lidocaine plasters, and capsaicin high concentration patches in specialized setting) for peripheral neuropathic pain, and sustained release tramadol (see Table 5.2 for official approvals for use).

Modified from Finnerup et al. (2015) and Moisset et al. (2020).

refer him to a specialized setting (therapeutic options may then include botulinum toxin A, noninvasive brain neurostimulation, or spinal cord stimulation).

KEY POINTS TO REMEMBER

- Diabetic painful neuropathy affects 15–35% of patients with diabetes and is more prevalent in type II diabetes. Risks may be enhanced by alcohol use.
- The initial management of diabetic neuropathy focuses on glycemic control and lifestyle measures.
- The first-line therapeutic options for painful diabetic neuropathic pain include FDA-approved gabapentin, pregabalin, and duloxetine.

- Other first-line treatments include tricyclic antidepressants.
- Second-line treatments for peripheral neuropathic pain in adults include, if pain area is limited, 5% lidocaine plasters and capsaicin high-concentration patches (in specialized settings).
- Other second-line drugs include sustained release tramadol (with careful monitoring).

Further Reading

Attal N, Bouhassira D. Advances in the treatment of neuropathic pain. *Curr Opin Neurol.* 2021;34(5):631–637.

Karlsson P, Gylfadottir SS, Andersen ST, et al. Painful and non-painful diabetic neuropathy, diagnostic challenges and implications for future management. *Brain.* 2021;144:1632–1645.

Sloan G, Selvarajah D, Tesfaye S. Pathogenesis, diagnosis and clinical management of diabetic sensorimotor peripheral neuropathy. *Nat Rev Endocrinol.* 2021;17:400–420.

Themistocleous AC, Ramirez JD, Shillo PR, et al. The Pain in Neuropathy Study (PiNS): A cross-sectional observational study determining the somatosensory phenotype of painful and painless diabetic neuropathy. *Pain.* 2016;157:1132–1145.

Truini A, Spallone V, Morganti R, et al.; Neuropathic Pain Special Interest Group of the Italian Society of Neurology. A cross-sectional study investigating frequency and features of definitely diagnosed diabetic painful polyneuropathy. *Pain.* 2018;159:2658–2666.

Ziegler D, Papanas N, Schnell O, et al. Current concepts in the management of diabetic polyneuropathy. *J Diabetes Investig.* 2021;12:464–475.

6 Painful Legs and Diabetes (2)

Nadine Attal and Didier Bouhassira

A 58-year-old woman with a long history of smoking and type II diabetes necessitating insulin therapy for several years complains of pain in the lower limbs, which started 2 years ago. Pain is often severe (7/10) and does not respond to conventional analgesics. It is described as deep aching and cramping particularly at walking but disappears after a few minutes of rest and involves the calves. Examination shows reduced sensation to pinprick at the feet and absent distal arterial pulses. Electromyography (EMG) shows an axonal neuropathy of the lower limbs. Considering the context and intensity of pain, her physician proposes duloxetine 60 mg daily, which has U.S. Food and Drug Administration approval for diabetic painful neuropathy. She has now received this treatment for more than 1 month and tolerates it well, but she reports strictly no efficacy.

What do you do now?

This woman with insulin-dependent diabetes reports chronic pain at the feet. A clinical examination shows reduced pinprick sensation at the feet, and EMG shows signs of axonal neuropathy. She has diabetic neuropathy. However, the outstanding question is whether her diabetic neuropathy is responsible for her pain.

You should pay particular attention to this woman's pain quality triggering factors and associated symptoms. You may ask her to fill out a screening neuropathic questionnaire (see Chapter 1). There is no burning, cold, or electric shocks. Rather, she describes her pain as deep aching and cramping. Her score on the LANSS is 3, which is lower than the cutoff value (≥ 12) for neuropathic pain (Figure 6.1).

Her leg pain is triggered by walking and disappears after a few minutes of rest. This is typical of claudication symptoms. Her pain involves the calves but not the feet. Physical examination shows vasomotor changes at the feet and legs and absent distal arterial pulses. Arterial Doppler and then angiography should be conducted. These examinations confirmed the presence of severe peripheral arterial disease. This woman finally underwent surgical revascularization. Recovery was total, and duloxetine could be gradually stopped.

Frequent causes of pain in the lower limbs linked with diabetes include other types of neuropathic pains (see Chapter 5) and nociceptive pains due mainly to ischemia related to peripheral arterial disease (Box 6.1). Importantly, most diabetic neuropathies are not painful or mainly induce paresthesia (e.g., tingling and numbness). Indeed, although diabetic neuropathy concerns up to 50% of patients with diabetes, neuropathic pain affects a fraction of patients with diabetic neuropathy (25–50%). This means that in many cases, diabetic patients have insensate neuropathy or that their pain is unrelated to the neuropathy. Furthermore, patients with painful and painless diabetic neuropathies generally have similar sensory deficits at the lower limbs, the main difference being the presence of brush evoked pain (allodynia), which is more common in painful patients, and EMG cannot discriminate between painful and painless neuropathies. Hence, particular attention should be paid to the pain quality, distribution, and aggravating factors. This case illustrates the relevance of screening neuropathic questionnaires in routine to discriminate neuropathic from nonneuropathic pains in diabetic patients even if the context orients toward diabetic painful neuropathy.

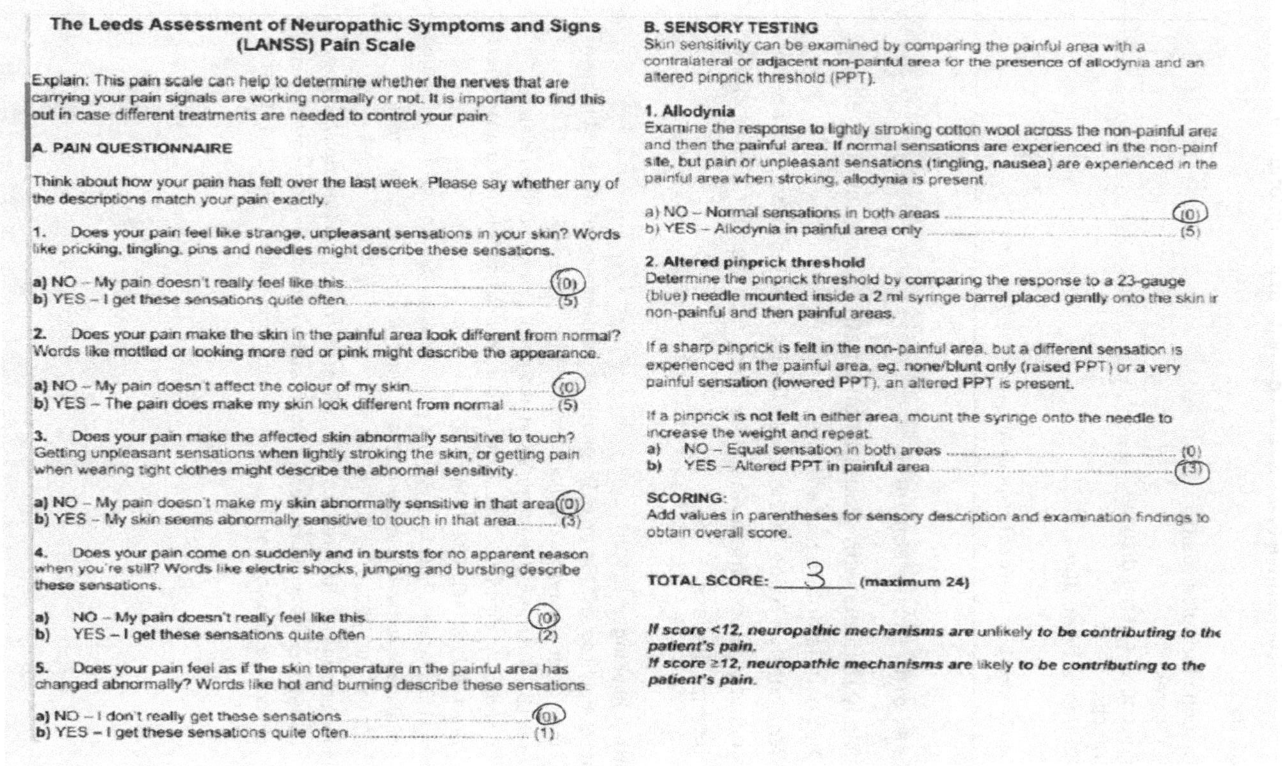

The Leeds Assessment of Neuropathic Symptoms and Signs (LANSS) Pain Scale

Explain: This pain scale can help to determine whether the nerves that are carrying your pain signals are working normally or not. It is important to find this out in case different treatments are needed to control your pain

A. PAIN QUESTIONNAIRE

Think about how your pain has felt over the last week. Please say whether any of the descriptions match your pain exactly.

1. Does your pain feel like strange, unpleasant sensations in your skin? Words like pricking, tingling, pins and needles might describe these sensations.

a) NO – My pain doesn't really feel like this .... (0)
b) YES – I get these sensations quite often .... (5)

2. Does your pain make the skin in the painful area look different from normal? Words like mottled or looking more red or pink might describe the appearance.

a) NO – My pain doesn't affect the colour of my skin .... (0)
b) YES – The pain does make my skin look different from normal .... (5)

3. Does your pain make the affected skin abnormally sensitive to touch? Getting unpleasant sensations when lightly stroking the skin, or getting pain when wearing tight clothes might describe the abnormal sensitivity.

a) NO – My pain doesn't make my skin abnormally sensitive in that area (0)
b) YES – My skin seems abnormally sensitive to touch in that area .... (3)

4. Does your pain come on suddenly and in bursts for no apparent reason when you're still? Words like electric shocks, jumping and bursting describe these sensations.

a) NO – My pain doesn't really feel like this .... (0)
b) YES – I get these sensations quite often .... (2)

5. Does your pain feel as if the skin temperature in the painful area has changed abnormally? Words like hot and burning describe these sensations.

a) NO – I don't really get these sensations .... (0)
b) YES – I get these sensations quite often .... (1)

B. SENSORY TESTING

Skin sensitivity can be examined by comparing the painful area with a contralateral or adjacent non-painful area for the presence of allodynia and an altered pinprick threshold (PPT).

1. Allodynia

Examine the response to lightly stroking cotton wool across the non-painful area and then the painful area. If normal sensations are experienced in the non-painful site, but pain or unpleasant sensations (tingling, nausea) are experienced in the painful area when stroking, allodynia is present.

a) NO – Normal sensations in both areas .... (0)
b) YES – Allodynia in painful area only .... (5)

2. Altered pinprick threshold

Determine the pinprick threshold by comparing the response to a 23-gauge (blue) needle mounted inside a 2 ml syringe barrel placed gently onto the skin in non-painful and then painful areas.

If a sharp pinprick is felt in the non-painful area, but a different sensation is experienced in the painful area, eg. none/blunt only (raised PPT) or a very painful sensation (lowered PPT), an altered PPT is present.

If a pinprick is not felt in either area, mount the syringe onto the needle to increase the weight and repeat.

a) NO – Equal sensation in both areas .... (0)
b) YES – Altered PPT in painful area .... (3)

SCORING:

Add values in parentheses for sensory description and examination findings to obtain overall score.

TOTAL SCORE: ___3___ (maximum 24)

If score <12, neuropathic mechanisms are unlikely to be contributing to the patient's pain.
If score ≥12, neuropathic mechanisms are likely to be contributing to the patient's pain.

FIGURE 6.1 Score obtained by the patient on the LANSS, a screening questionnaire for neuropathic pain (see Chapter 1). Neuropathic pain is likely for a cutoff value ≥ 12 on this scale. The score obtained is 3, which means that neuropathic pain is unlikely.

KEY POINTS TO REMEMBER

- Many patients with diabetic neuropathy have pain in the feet, but pain is not necessarily neuropathic.
- Nociceptive pains in the lower limbs in relation with diabetes include ulcers, infections, bedsores, arthropathy, and peripheral arterial disease.

Further Reading

Attal N, Bouhassira D, Baron R. Diagnosis and assessment of neuropathic pain through questionnaires. *Lancet Neurol.* 2018;17:456–466.

Jensen TS, Karlsson P, Gylfadottir SS, et al. Painful and non-painful diabetic neuropathy, diagnostic challenges and implications for future management. *Brain.* 2021;8(144):1632–1645.

Sloan G, Selvarajah D, Tesfaye S. Pathogenesis, diagnosis and clinical management of diabetic sensorimotor peripheral neuropathy. *Nat Rev Endocrinol.* 2021;17:400–420.

Themistocleous AC, Ramirez JD, Shillo PR, et al. The Pain in Neuropathy Study (PiNS): A cross-sectional observational study determining the somatosensory phenotype of painful and painless diabetic neuropathy. *Pain.* 2016;157:1132–1145.

7   Groin Pain After Hernia Repair

Nadine Attal and Didier Bouhassira

A 32-year-old construction worker was operated on for left inguinal hernia (open surgery) a few months ago. Immediately after surgery, he started feeling intense pain described as hot/burning in the scar site and surrounding area in the groin, scrotum, and upper thigh. Eight months after surgery, groin pain has persisted, although more moderate (6/10) and mainly reported as lancinating or deep aching. Examination of the painful area discloses mild pinprick and cold deficit compared to the contralateral side, allodynia to brush, as well as red skin and swelling. He was first treated with NSAIDs, paracetamol, and then codeine paracetamol combination without efficacy. Duloxetine, gabapentin, pregabalin, and tramadol were subsequently proposed, but the patient refused these treatments because of their potential risks of somnolence and sexual side effects. He resumed his professional activity and states that he prefers to avoid any systemic medications because he does not want to risk any bothersome side effects that may cause prejudice to his work.

What do you do now?

This patient, who underwent surgery for hernia repair, suffers from chronic groin pain (more than 3 months). Pain was not present before surgery and started soon after his operation. It may be considered as postsurgical.

This patient's spontaneous pain is mainly described as shooting, but screening questionnaires may be helpful to further detect whether pain is neuropathic. His score on the DN4 questionnaire is 7/10, which suggests neuropathic pain (see Chapter 1). The area of pain in the scar and surrounding area corresponds to the surgical site and is compatible with a neuroanatomical territory (the genitals and upper part of the thigh, corresponding to ilioinguinal, iliohypogastric, or genitofemoral nerves). Clinical examination (best conducted by comparison with the normal contralateral side, Chapter 1) discloses mild pinprick and cold (thermoalgesic) deficit in the painful area, allodynia to brush, and vasomotor changes, which are common after surgery. This fits the diagnostic of postsurgical neuropathic pain. Complementary examinations such as electromyography, which is difficult to conduct in this area, are not mandatory.

This patient was reluctant to take oral drugs because of potential side effects. His pain did not respond to conventional analgesics including weak opioids, which is not surprising given its neuropathic mechanisms. The best approach is to propose topical treatments because the area of pain is delineated and restricted (Chapter 28). He was treated with off-label 5% lidocaine plasters (one plaster during 12 hours to cover the painful area). The immediate efficacy was moderate but judged acceptable. After a few months, the patient noticed consistent improvement in his pain. He now mainly feels paresthesia in the painful area. This suggests that there was spontaneous recovery 1 year after surgery, which is the most common situation.

Groin hernia repair represents one of the major causes of surgery, and persistent pain is observed in approximately 10% of cases (of which 30% are neuropathic). Neuroma formation may play a role, but nerve damage can also occur from manipulation, traction, thermal damage during surgery, or inflammation due to a fibrotic mesh reaction after surgery. Other common causes of postsurgical neuropathic pain include thoracotomy, mastectomy, knee/hip replacement, cholecystectomy, and varicose vein stripping (Figure 7.1).

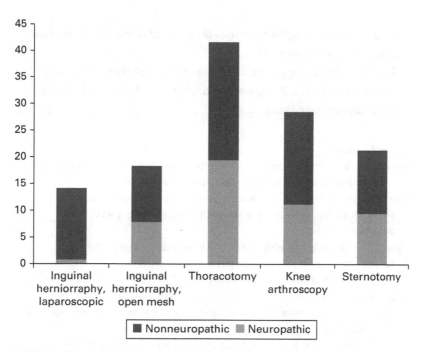

FIGURE 7.1 Prevalence of postsurgical inguinal pain (and neuropathic pain assessed with the DN4 interview, cutoff ≥3/7 for detection of neuropathic pain) after herniorraphy and other major surgeries at 6 months in a French multicenter prospective study (2014).

Therapeutic management is similar to that of other neuropathic pains, but if pain is refractory to conventional medical management, surgical management (laparoscopic retroperitoneal neurectomy) has sometimes been found to be beneficial in the case of persistent pain after hernia repair.

KEY POINTS TO REMEMBER

- Postsurgical pain is commonly neuropathic.
- Main risk factors include preoperative and acute postoperative pain, including acute neuropathic pain; preoperative opioid use; the nature of surgery; and psychosocial or cognitive factors.
- Pain is typically described as neuropathic and commonly associated with allodynia and vasomotor or sudomotor changes (e.g., red skin and swelling). It is situated in the neuroanatomical

area corresponding to the injured nerve, sometimes in the scar site and surrounding skin area.

- Therapeutic management is similar to that of other peripheral neuropathic pains. If the area of pain is small, the best choice includes topical agents.

Further Reading

Aasvang EK, Gmaehle E, Hansen JB, et al. Predictive risk factors for persistent postherniotomy pain. *Anesthesiology*. 2010;112:957–969.

Chen DC, Hiatt JR, Amid PK. Operative management of refractory neuropathic inguinodynia by a laparoscopic retroperitoneal approach. *JAMA Surg*. 2013;148(10):962–967.

Dualé C, Ouchchane L, Schoeffler P, EDONIS Investigating Group, Dubray C. Neuropathic aspects of persistent postsurgical pain: A French multicenter survey with a 6-month prospective follow-up. *J Pain*. 2014;15:24.e1–24.e20.

Haroutounian S, Nikolajsen L, Finnerup NB, Jensen TS. The neuropathic component in persistent postsurgical pain: A systematic literature review. *Pain*. 2013;154:95–102.

Jensen EK, Ringsted TK, Bischoff JM, et al. A national center for persistent severe pain after groin hernia repair: Five-year prospective data. *Medicine*. 2019;98:e16600.

Kehlet H, Jensen TS, Woolf CJ. Persistent postsurgical pain: Risk factors and prevention. *Lancet*. 2006;367:1618–1625.

Martinez V, Ammar SB, Judet T, et al. Risk factors predictive of chronic postsurgical neuropathic pain: The value of the iliac crest bone harvest model. *Pain*. 2012;153:1478–1483.

8 Pain and Paresthesia of the Hand

Anne-Priscille Trouvin

A 42-year-old woman with rheumatoid arthritis (RA) treated by methotrexate consults her doctor for pain in the right hand. At her last visit 3 months ago with her rheumatologist, her disease activity score (DAS-28) was 2.4, which is in favor of remission, and treatment was maintained with a weekly dosage of 15 mg and intermittent corticosteroids. One month ago, she started feeling tingling and moderate pain in her right hand and wrist, which were aggravated at night, and she noticed mild swelling. Believing she was having a flare of RA, she self-medicated with low doses of corticosteroids and paracetamol. These treatments did not change her symptoms, which increased day after day with pain radiating to the forearm. She now describes tingling, pins and needles, and sometimes burning pain at the right wrist and palmar area of the thumb and index finger, extending to the forearm. Clinical examination shows no apparent sensory deficit, no muscle weakness, and no atrophy. Percussion of the median nerve at the wrist, but not forced flexion of the wrist, tends to induce paresthesia. There are no other painful joints.

What do you do now?

This woman with RA has tingling, pins and needles (paresthesia), and sometimes burning pain at the right wrist and palmar area of the thumb and index finger, which corresponds to the median nerve territory. Paresthesia is increased by percussion of the median nerve at the wrist (Tinel sign). The symptoms and results of clinical examination are consistent with the diagnosis of carpal tunnel syndrome (compression of the median nerve at the wrist) associated with RA. RA may be associated with various nerve complications, but entrapment neuropathies are the most frequent (estimated prevalence of 10%; twofold increased risk compared to the general adult population).

This diagnosis generally does not necessitate complementary investigations if the clinical picture is typical. In atypical cases or when symptoms are severe, complementary investigations may be necessary, such as nerve conduction studies, magnetic resonance imaging, or ultrasonography of the median nerve (Figure 8.1). Now you need to search for a cause or risk factor (Table 8.1). Are her symptoms related to a flare of RA, or do they come

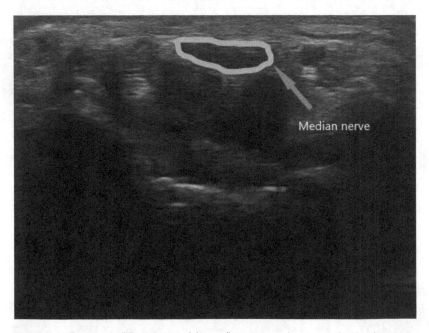

Median nerve

FIGURE 8.1 Transverse sliding patterns of the median nerve on ultrasonography showing pathological enlargement of the nerve at the wrist.

TABLE 8.1   Description, Risk Factors, and Diagnosis of Carpal Tunnel Syndrome

Description and clinical maneuvers to confirm diagnosis	Initial symptoms: intermittent nocturnal paresthesia/dysesthesia in the median nerve territory (palmar surface of the wrist, thumb, index finger, middle finger, external part of the fourth finger); may involve the entire palm, rarely above wrist Progression: continuous symptoms at daytime, numbness, loss of sensation, thenar muscle weakness, muscle atrophy Pain (±50%): may extend to the forearm Tinel sign: percussion of median nerve at the wrist to produce paresthesia (sensitivity, 38–100%; specificity, 55–100%) Phalen maneuver: forced flexion of the wrist (1 mn) to produce paresthesia (sensitivity, 42–85%; specificity, 54–98%)
Risk factors	Rheumatoid arthritis (compression by synovitis/tenosynovitis, articular malalignments) Hypothyroidism Diabetes mellitus Obesity Pregnancy Menopause
Diagnosis	Mainly clinical (paresthesia and/or pain in the median nerve territory ± maneuvers) Complementary investigations mainly for severe symptoms: Nerve conduction studies: objective measurement of the nerve but imperfect sensitivity/specificity Magnetic resonance imaging: if suspicion of synovitis/tenosynovitis Ultrasonography of the median nerve: if suspicion of local cause of compression

Adapted from Padua et al. (2016).

from another condition? Assessment of the wrist and search for signs of tenderness, swelling, or nodules (suggestive of synovitis or tenosynovitis) may require rheumatologist advice. Biological tests should search for diabetes mellitus (especially for this patient receiving corticosteroids), hypothyroidism, and pregnancy. Differential diagnosis should be excluded, particularly cervical radiculopathy (the latter generally includes cervical and brachial pain extending to the hand and reduced or absent tendon reflexes at the upper limb). Neck imaging and electromyography may confirm the diagnosis but are not mandatory. Other differential diagnoses include polyneuropathies (symptoms are bilateral and usually affect the lower limbs first) and osteoarthritis (no neuropathic symptoms).

After diagnostic setup, you may propose rest, education (to achieve a change of habits in wrist movements and heavy carrying), ergonomic work tools, splinting (but its duration is not codified), and local corticosteroids. Antineuropathic treatments are not necessary, particularly as entrapment syndromes are seldom very painful (except sometimes after surgery, see Chapter 7). If carpal tunnel syndrome is caused by RA flare, you should ask for specialist advice to adjust the treatment of RA. You may refer this patient for surgical treatment (decompression of the carpal tunnel by transection of the transverse carpal ligament) in (rare) cases of refractory pain or motor symptoms with functional impairment.

In this woman, nerve conduction study confirmed the diagnostic of entrapment neuropathy of the median nerve at the wrists. She had no signs of flare, but biological screening evidenced type I hypothyroidism, which necessitated thyroid hormone therapy. She was first treated by splinting and then corticosteroid injections with excellent efficacy. Surgical intervention was not required.

KEY POINTS TO REMEMBER

- Carpal tunnel syndrome is mainly a clinical diagnosis based on accurate and comprehensive clinical history with exclusion of differential diagnosis.
- Carpal tunnel syndrome is seldom painful and most patients mainly complain of paresthesia (e.g., tingling). Antineuropathic

drug treatments such as antidepressants or antiepileptics are generally not necessary.
- Complementary explorations are not always mandatory. Nerve conduction studies may provide objective confirmation of decreased sensory and motor conduction of the median nerve at the wrist. Imaging particularly using ultrasound can help when there is strong suspicion of a local cause of compression.
- Risk factors such as diabetes mellitus and hypothyroidism should be searched.
- Treatment includes rest, splinting, and local corticosteroid injections. In refractory cases or when there is motor involvement, surgical decompression is indicated.

Further Reading

Agarwal V, Singh R, Wiclaf, et al. A clinical, electrophysiological, and pathological study of neuropathy in rheumatoid arthritis. *Clin Rheumatol.* 2008;27:841–844.

DeQuattro K., Imboden JB. Neurologic manifestations of rheumatoid arthritis. *Rheum Dis Clin North Am.* 2017;43(4):561–571.

Muramatsu K, Tanaka H, Taguchi T. Peripheral neuropathies of the forearm and hand in rheumatoid arthritis: Diagnosis and options for treatment. *Rheumatol Int.* 2008;28:951–957.

Padua L, Coraci D, Erra C, et al. Carpal tunnel syndrome: Clinical features, diagnosis, and management. *Lancet Neurol.* 2016;15(12):1273–1284.

Shiri R. Arthritis as a risk factor for carpal tunnel syndrome: A meta-analysis. *Scand J Rheumatol.* 2016;45:339–346.

9 Pain After Surgery for Hand Fracture

Manon Sendel, Janne Gierthmühlen,
and Ralf Baron

A 37-year-old woman presents with persistent pain
3 months after surgery for radial fracture. She states
that pain never subsided after surgery and even
got worse after starting physiotherapy. In addition
to a stinging sensation in the former surgical area,
she also describes a burning pain of changing
intensity in her whole left hand, including all fingers,
accompanied by an increased sensitivity to touch.
Range of movement is greatly impaired. Furthermore,
she noticed a swelling and reddish-blue color of the
whole hand, including the fingers. Wearing a glove is
not possible due to the swelling as well as sensitivity.
She consulted again her orthopedist, who rules out
any pseudarthrosis, problems regarding implanted
screws and plates, infection, or vascular pathology.

What do you do now?

This woman reports persisting persistent pain, discoloration, edema, and impaired range of motion after surgery for hand fracture. Her orthopedist ruled out pseudarthrosis, infection, or vascular pathology. The temporal relationship of her pain with surgery, pain characteristics, area of pain, examination, and inspection are essential for the diagnosis.

Although this woman had pain before surgery, there was a consistent change in the character of her pain after surgery. Hence, her pain may be considered as postsurgical. Now her pain characteristics include burning, stinging sensation, and evoked pain to touch (allodynia), which are characteristics of neuropathic pain. However, contrary to "classical" neuropathic pains, her pain is not localized to a dermatoma (e.g., the median nerve) but, rather, extends to the whole left hand, including all fingers. She also reports some coarse black hair growing on her hand, which she cut off. At inspection, her right hand is swollen with elapsed joint furrows. The skin on her right hand looks plump and glossy with a light reddish-livid skin coloration. At physical examination, her hand is very sensitive to touch, and she experiences pain when pressure is applied to her small finger joints. The palm is sweaty. She cannot close her right hand to make a fist and is not able to reach her thumb with her middle or ring finger.

This clinical picture typically corresponds to complex regional pain syndrome (CRPS), formerly called algodystrophy. The area of pain, which extends beyond a neuroanatomical area to cover the whole hand in a "glove"-like distribution, is poorly consistent with a postsurgical nerve lesion. CRPS is characterized by somatosensory abnormalities and often occurs after surgery. Other events responsible are major trauma, such as bone fracture of the hand, or minor trauma, such as sprained ankle, and sometimes stroke and myocardiac infarction; some conditions are idiopathic. CRPS is two to four times more prevalent in women than men. Autonomic nervous system, genetic factors, depression, and post-traumatic stress disorder might play a role or increase the risk of CRPS.

CRPS is mainly a clinical diagnostic (Table 9.1), but magnetic resonance imaging or three-phase bone scintigraphy (3PBS) may contribute to the diagnosis. In particular, 3PBS may show a characteristic uptake pattern in the late (bone metabolism) phase in the affected limb (diffuse osteoporosis with patchy demineralization, especially of the periarticular regions, and

TABLE 9.1 **Revised Budapest Clinical Diagnostic Criteria for CRPS**

1. Continuing pain, disproportionate to the inciting event

2. Must report at least one symptom in three of the four following categories:

Sensory	Hyperesthesia and/or allodynia
Vasomotor	Temperature asymmetry and/or skin color changes and/or skin color asymmetry
Sudomotor/edema	Edema and/or sweating changes and/or sweating asymmetry
Motor/trophic	Decreased range of motion and/or motor dysfunction (weakness, tremor, dystonia) and/or trophic changes (hair, nail, skin)

3. Must display at least one sign at time of evaluation in two or more of the following categories:

Sensory	Evidence of hyperalgesia (to pinprick) and/or allodynia (to light touch and/or deep somatic pressure and/or joint movement)
Vasomotor	Evidence of temperature asymmetry and/or skin color changes and/or skin color asymmetry
Sudomotor/edema	Evidence of edema and/or sweating changes and/or sweating asymmetry
Motor/trophic	Decreased range of motion and/or motor dysfunction (weakness, tremor, dystonia) and/or trophic changes (hair, nail, skin)

4. There is no other diagnosis that better explains the signs and symptoms

subperiosteal bone resorption) (Figure 9.1). However, sensitivity and specificity decrease after the first year of the disease; thus, a negative 3PBS does not rule out CRPS. Other tests in specialized centers include skin temperature measurements (showing temperature changes), quantitative sensory testing (showing hyperalgesia to pressure pain in approximately 70% of cases), and tests of sudomotor function (showing impaired sudomotor function).

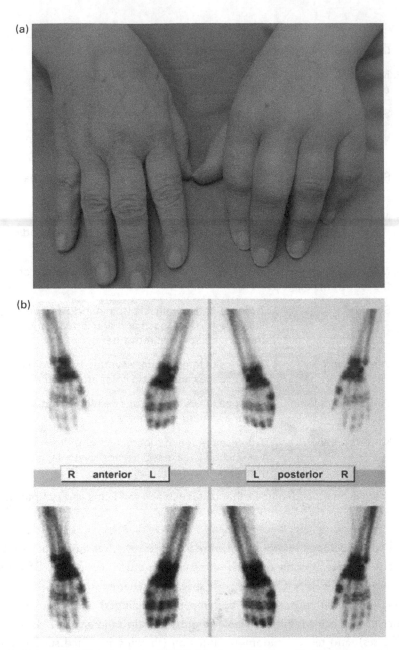

FIGURE 9.1 (*Top*) Clinical aspects of CRPS of the hand. (*Middle and bottom*) Results of three-phase bone scintigraphy in CRPS.

You should treat this woman as soon as the diagnosis is suspected (Table 9.2). The most urgent is to preserve and regain function of her affected limb. Hence, physiotherapy and occupational therapy should be started early, at least twice a week. Because symptoms of (neurogenic) inflammation are prominent, you may also try short-term corticosteroids (the benefit of nonsteroidal anti-inflammatory drugs is not well documented).

TABLE 9.2   **Proposed Treatment Recommendations for CRPS[a]**

Pharmacologic treatment	Oral antineuropathic drugs such as - Gabapentin 3 × 600–1200 mg/day - Pregabalin 2 × 75–300 mg/day - Amitriptyline 25–75 mg/day Consider bisphosphonates (e.g., alendronate p.o. 40 mg/day for 8 weeks)
Presence of inflammatory signs	Glucocorticoids (e.g., prednisolone p.o. 100 mg per day in descending regimen and tapering off over 2½ weeks)
Signs suggestive of severe sympathetic dysfunction (e.g., severe sudomotor or vasomotor changes)	Consider sympathetic blocks
Physical therapy	Also includes lymphatic drainage and graded motor imagery
Occupational therapy	Includes desensitization
Behavioral therapy	Encourages the patient coping and acceptance, treats comorbid depression, etc.
In case of refractory pain	Consider ketamine infusions Consider spinal cord stimulation
In case of focal dystonia	Consider intrathecal baclofen

[a]These treatment recommendations are adapted from German guidelines for diagnostic and therapy of complex regional pain syndrome and from authors' clinical experience (Gierthmühlen J, Binder A, Baron R. Mechanism-based treatment in complex regional pain syndromes. Nat Rev Neurol. 2014 Sep;10(9):518–28). There is no specific "CRPS" official indication for use; gabapentin, pregabalin, and amitriptyline are recommended for neuropathic pain (Chapter 2) and biphosphonates are approved for osteoporosis. Sympathetic blocks have no high-quality evidence confirming their efficacy in CRPS, and ketamine infusions have very weak evidence for efficacy (Chapter 40).

Other potential therapies include drugs effective for neuropathic pain such as gabapentinoids or antidepressants, although there is poor evidence for their efficacy in this context. Graded motor imagery and mirror therapy may be proposed by specialized physiotherapists (see Chapter 30). Sympathetic blocks might also be considered, but evidence regarding their efficacy remains very low (see Chapter 40). For refractory cases, transcranial magnetic stimulation, spinal cord stimulation, or dorsal root ganglion stimulation may be considered. Spinal cord stimulation in particular has been found to be effective based on controlled studies (see Chapter 44). Other less commonly proposed invasive options include intrathecal therapy with ziconotide or baclofen (see Chapter 45), particularly in the case of severe motor symptoms such as dystonia. In all cases, complementary treatments such as relaxation may be beneficial.

This woman was started on physiotherapy. Because physiotherapy was extremely painful initially, she was sent to an anesthesiologist, who performed regional analgesic blockade to facilitate the first rehabilitation sessions. After a few sessions, this treatment was stopped and she was advised to take strong analgesics (oral immediate-release morphine 10 mg) 1 hour before physiotherapy. Concomitantly, she received oral prednisone 60 mg per day during 15 days and then tapered off for the next 7 days. She progressively regained a better function of her hand, and her pain progressively decreased in severity. However, she still is in significant pain after 1 year. Hence, additional treatments such as spinal cord stimulation are being seriously considered by specialists.

KEY POINTS TO REMEMBER

- CRPS should be considered when a change of pain character (e.g., from dull to burning, etc.) and somatosensory abnormalities occur in combination with motor and autonomic abnormalities.
- CRPS is a clinical diagnosis. Additional diagnostic methods such as 3PBS can support the diagnosis, but the absence of typical results does not rule it out.

- Symptoms of CRPS and neuropathic pain often overlap. The most important difference is that in CRPS, pain is not limited to a certain innervation territory.
- Treatment should be preferably multimodal and may involve neuromodulating agents, physical/occupational therapy, psychological therapy, and, less commonly, corticosteroids and sympathetic nerve blocks.
- For refractory CRPS, spinal cord stimulation has the best level of evidence.

Further Reading

Cepeda MS, Lau J, Carr DB. Defining the therapeutic role of local anesthetic sympathetic blockade in complex regional pain syndrome: A narrative and systematic review. *Clin J Pain*. 2002;18(4):216–233.

Gierthmühlen J, Binder A, Baron R. Mechanism-based treatment in complex regional pain syndromes. *Nat Rev Neurol*. 2014;10(9):518–528.

Gierthmühlen J, Maier C, Baron R, et al.; German Research Network on Neuropathic Pain (DFNS) study group. Sensory signs in complex regional pain syndrome and peripheral nerve injury. *Pain*. 2012;153(4):765–774.

Goebel A, Birklein F, Brunner F, et al. The Valencia consensus-based adaptation of the IASP complex regional pain syndrome diagnostic criteria. *Pain*. 2021;162(9):2346–2348.

Harden NR, Bruehl S, Perez RSGM, et al. Validation of proposed diagnostic criteria (the "Budapest Criteria") for complex regional pain syndrome. *Pain*. 2010;150(2):268–274.

Wüppenhorst N, Maier C, Frettlöh J, Pennekamp W, Nicolas V. Sensitivity and specificity of 3-phase bone scintigraphy in the diagnosis of complex regional pain syndrome of the upper extremity. *Clin J Pain*. 2010;26(3):182–189.

10 Pain After Amputation

Nadine Attal and Didier Bouhassira

A 58-year-old man is referred for evaluation to your clinic because of left foot pain after mid-thigh amputation. The amputation occurred after he stepped on a land mine in Cambodia when he was 23 years old. His pain is worse in the missing foot, described as electric shocks and stabbing. He wears a prosthetic leg. Since the amputation, he has also suffered from post-traumatic stress disorder (PTSD), with nightmares and panic attacks. His pain has been poorly responsive to opioids and local nerve blocks, and gabapentin, pregabalin, and amitriptyline were not tolerated. He has also tried transcutaneous electrical nerve stimulation but states that it does not reduce his pain. He is reluctant to try additional oral medications.

What do you do now?

This patient reports severe foot pain after mid-thigh amputation. It is important to determine if his pain is situated in his stump (stump pain, generally described as electric shocks or evoked by gently tapping the stump), felt in his missing limb, or both. Here, pain predominates in the missing foot. It is mainly described as paroxysmal with electric shocks and stabbing pain. This fits the usual description of phantom limb pain. The latter may also be described as burning or cold, associated with paresthesia or dysesthesia, as is the case for other neuropathic pains (Table 10.1).

This patient previously received multiple therapies for his phantom limb pain (tricyclic antidepressants, pregabalin, gabapentin, opioids, and transcutaneous electrical nerve stimulation) but did not tolerate them or they were poorly effective. He is seeking other therapeutic options.

TABLE 10.1 **Main Differences Between Phantom Limb Pain and Stump Pain**

	Phantom Limb Pain	Stump Pain
Area of pain	Pain felt in the missing limb	Pain felt in the stump
Clinical characteristics	Paroxysmal pain (electric shocks), burning pain, tingling, no allodynia	Paroxysmal pain, burning pain, mechanical allodynia of the stump (gently tapping increases the pain)
Main mechanisms	Neuronal plasticity and reorganization of the somatosensory cortex triggered by peripheral mechanisms	Ectopic activity generated in the stump neuroma
Therapeutic management	Oral antineuropathic drugs (pregabalin, gabapentin, duloxetine, tricyclic antidepressants, tramadol as second line and strong opioids as last choice) Physical therapy (prosthesis with somatosensory input, proprioceptive training, mirror therapy, motor imagery training)	Oral antineuropathic drugs Topical drugs (e.g., lidocaine plasters, capsaicin high-concentration patches in specialized setting) Transcutaneous electrical nerve stimulation

Since this patient suffers from PTSD, you should first ask him to consult a psychiatrist for potential pharmacological (e.g., selective serotonin reuptake inhibitor antidepressants) and/or nonpharmacological (e.g., eye movement desensitization and reprocessing [EMDR]) therapy for PTSD. You may also refer him to a specialized physiotherapy clinic for proprioceptive training, mirror therapy, or related techniques (motor imagery training and immersive virtual reality based on mirror therapy) (Chapter 30). The latter are based on visual feedback of one's intact limb in a mirror (mirror therapy) or aim to transpose the movements made by the remaining limb into movements of a virtual limb (virtual reality), thus providing the impression of viewing the amputation limb.

This patient was started on paroxetine 20 mg per day, which contributed to relieve his stress, and consulted a psychiatrist for EMDR. He then received mirror limb therapy by a physiotherapist, which improved his pain by 50%.

Positive sensations referred to a missing limb after amputation have been reported since the 16th century, with the French surgeon Ambroise Paré first describing this post-amputation phenomenon. Amputations worldwide are often related to traumatic injury caused by accidents or conflicts (e.g., land mines), whereas in Western countries they are mainly due to diabetes mellitus or vascular diseases (gangrene), less commonly trauma or cancer, and rarely congenital malformations. Although phantom sensations are reported by almost all amputees (with modifications of perception of the limb over time, including telescoping—that is, feeling that the phantom limb gradually shrinks over time), these sensations have little impact on quality of life, contrary to phantom limb pain.

Phantom limb pain corresponds to pain felt in the amputated limb and has also been reported after mastectomy, enucleation, or tooth avulsion (phantom tooth). Pain may occur soon after surgery and tends to decrease within the first 6 months, but it may also be delayed and persist for years. It is often reported distally in the missing limb (foot, toes, hand, or fingers), probably because of the larger representation of distal body parts in the somatosensory cortex. Risk factors include preamputation pain (more than 60% of patients with phantom limb pain describe similar symptoms as their preoperative pain), phantom sensation, stump pain, diabetes, and psychosocial factors (passive coping, catastrophizing, and poor social environment). Mechanisms probably involve maladaptive plasticity and reorganization of the somatosensory cortex (a process by which neighboring regions of the area representing the lost limb expand along the cortical map, the degree of which generally correlates with the severity of pain), but these central mechanisms are generally maintained by peripheral mechanisms (ectopic activity generated in the stump neuroma, and responsible for stump pain). This explains why many patients report both stump and phantom limb pain and why the use of a prosthesis providing somatosensory input is probably protective, contrary to purely cosmetic prosthetic legs. Conventional therapeutic approaches, akin to other neuropathic pains, include duloxetine, tricyclic antidepressants, pregabalin, gabapentin, tramadol as second line, while topical agents (e.g., 5 % lidocaine plasters, high concentration capsaicin patches, botulinum toxin A) are only suitable for stump pain. Strong opioids may be proposed as last choice for refractory cases. Specific therapeutic approaches include mirror therapy, virtual reality, proprioceptive training, and prosthetic and surgical approaches generally combined with rehabilitation techniques including targeted muscle reinnervation to restore physiological continuity.

KEY POINTS TO REMEMBER

- After amputations, most patients experience phantom limb, and a subgroup may experience phantom limb pain.
- Mechanisms include maladaptive plasticity, reorganization of the somatosensory cortex, and ectopic discharges from the stump neuroma.
- Conventional therapeutic approaches are similar to those of other neuropathic pains and include tricyclic antidepressants, duloxetine, pregabalin, gabapentin, tramadol, and topical agents (for stump pain), while strong opioids are only recommended for refractory cases.
- Other therapeutic approaches include mirror therapy, virtual reality, proprioceptive training, and prosthetic and surgical approaches generally combined with rehabilitation techniques including targeted muscle reinnervation to restore physiological continuity.

Further Reading

Erlenwein J, Diers M, Ernst J, Schulz F, Petzke F. Clinical updates on phantom limb pain. *Pain Rep*. 2021;6(1):e888.

Giraux P, Sirigu A. Illusory movements of the paralyzed limb restore motor cortex activity. *NeuroImage*. 2003;20(Suppl 1):S107–S111.

Giummarra MJ, Moseley GL. Phantom limb pain and bodily awareness: Current concepts and future directions. *Curr Opin Anaesthesiol*. 2011;24(5):524–531.

Limakatso K, Bedwell GJ, Madden VJ, Parker R. The prevalence and risk factors for phantom limb pain in people with amputations: A systematic review and meta-analysis. *PLoS One*. 2020;15(10):e0240431.

Ramachandran VS, Altschuler EL. The use of visual feedback, in particular mirror visual feedback, in restoring brain function. *Brain*. 2009;132(Pt 7):1693–1710.

11 Pain and Breast Cancer Surgery

Nadine Attal and Didier Bouhassira

A 52-year-old woman with type II diabetes was operated on 2 years ago for right mastectomy and lymph node dissection preceded by radiotherapy. She receives tamoxifen, an antiaromatase treatment. She reports persistent severe pain at the right shoulder, mild pain induced by pressure on the breast, and diffuse widespread pain. She also feels anxious and has sleep disorders. Her shoulder pain started before surgery and after radiotherapy. It is described as cramping, lancinating, increased by movement, and decreased by rest. Examination discloses reduced range of shoulder motion and hypoesthesia to tactile stimuli in the breast and axilla. A physician concluded that she suffered from post-mastectomy neuropathic pain and prescribed pregabalin up to 100 mg TID, but she states that pregabalin has no efficacy and that she gained weight with this treatment. She wants to know whether she can stop pregabalin and whether other treatments would be appropriate for her pain.

What do you do now?

This woman underwent surgery for breast cancer, radiotherapy, and antiaromatase treatment. She now suffers from persistent shoulder pain (on the site of surgery), moderate pressure-evoked pain in the breast area, and widespread pain. Her worst pain is in the shoulder. A physician concluded that she has neuropathic pain because of her medical history (surgery), area of pain, and the fact that pain is present in an area of sensory deficit.

Does this woman have postsurgical neuropathic pain? Her pain started after radiotherapy and was present before surgery, but it tended to increase after antiaromatase therapy. Thus, pain is not postsurgical. Her worse pain is in the shoulder, aggravated by shoulder movement and decreased by rest. It is described as cramping and lancinating. There is no burning, electric shocks, evoked pain, or paresthesia—hence no neuropathic characteristics (you may be helped by a screening questionnaire; here the score at the DN4 interview was 1/7, which seems to rule out neuropathic pain (see Chapter 1). Examination discloses sensory deficit in the breast and axilla and reduced range of motion of the shoulder.

Thus, in this woman who underwent breast surgery from cancer, pain does not result from breast surgery and has no neuropathic characteristics. The presence of sensory deficit in the axilla suggests that there was nerve impairment because of surgery, which is common (the nerve involved generally corresponding to the intercostobrachial nerve), but this nerve lesion was not responsible for her pain. Of note, most surgical nerve lesions are not painful, and only a small proportion induce neuropathic pain.

You have probably already suspected that this woman suffers from adhesive capsulitis or frozen shoulder. Here, the diagnosis of adhesive capsulitis of the shoulder enhanced by radiotherapy was confirmed by a rheumatologist. Of note, this woman had diabetes, which probably increased her risk of adhesive capsulitis. Regarding her other symptoms, her mild pressure-evoked pain in the breast area may be due to radiation tissue damage, and her widespread pain may be related to antiaromatase therapy because these antihormone treatments sometimes induce widespread pain.

For this woman, you should first taper off pregabalin, which not only was ineffective but also increased her weight; this should be conducted gradually, if she has received this treatment for several months, by removing 75 mg every 3–7 days until complete cessation of the drug. You should also propose nonsteroidal anti-inflammatory drugs such as ibuprofen (800 mg per day) and physical therapy. Finally, because of her anxiety, you may ask for a psychologist's or a psychiatrist's advice. It is not necessary to treat her other pain symptoms because they are mild and have little impact on her quality of life.

This woman tapered off pregabalin gradually, which was stopped after 3 weeks. Concomitantly, she started ibuprofen 800 mg per day for 3 weeks combined with physical therapy. The latter was judged difficult and painful initially, but paracetamol 1 g was added 1 hour before each physical session and this was helpful for decreasing induced pain. After 1 month, her pain is no longer present. Pain has been reported in 20–50% of women after mastectomy (generally referred to as post- mastectomy pain) or cosmetic breast surgery (Table 11.1). Patients with breast cancer surgery, radiotherapy, and chemotherapy are at risk for several types of neuropathic pain, but nociceptive pain after mastectomy with or without radiotherapy is even

TABLE 11.1 **Common Causes of Pain After Mastectomy for Breast Cancer**

Classification	Pain Mechanisms	Pain Areas
Neuropathic pain	Surgical lesion (generally the intercostobrachial nerve due to lymph node dissection)	Axilla, inner surface of arm, breast, anterolateral chest wall
	Brachial plexopathy (radiation therapy)	Arm, breast, axilla
	Painful neuropathy (chemotherapy)	Distal extremities (feet, hands)
	Epiduritis (bone metastases)	Variable: generally presents as radicular pain, sometimes central pain (due to myelopathy)
Nociceptive pain	Hormonal depletion (antiaromatase therapy)	Widespread pain or joint pain
	Tissue fibrosis (radiation therapy)	Breast, arm, chest
	Adhesive capsulitis (radiation therapy, surgery)	Shoulder, arm
	Myofascial pain (surgery)	Shoulder, arm, chest
	Rotator cuff injury (surgery, lymphedema, radiation)	Shoulder
	Bone metastasis	Variable

more common. Particularly after a certain age, these women may also have chronic pain independently of surgery or radiotherapy.

KEY POINTS TO REMEMBER

- Pain is common after mastectomy and may be neuropathic (generally related to an injury of the intercostobrachial nerve) or nociceptive (generally related to soft tissue injury).
- Risk factors include young age, high BMI, lymph node dissection, preoperative pain, and radiotherapy.
- It may be difficult to differentiate distinct pain mechanisms when several types of pains are present in the same neuroanatomical territory, and this may need screening neuropathic questionnaires.

Further Reading

Andersen KG, Duriaud HM, Jensen HE, Kroman N, Kehlet H. Predictive factors for the development of persistent pain after breast cancer surgery. *Pain*. 2015;156(12):2413–2422.

Date A, Rahman L. Frozen shoulder: Overview of clinical presentation and review of the current evidence base for management strategies. *Future Sci OA*. 2020;6(10):FSO647.

Habib AS, Kertai MD, Cooter M, Greenup RA, Hwang S. Risk factors for severe acute pain and persistent pain after surgery for breast cancer: A prospective observational study. *Reg Anesth Pain Med*. 2019;44(2):192–199.

Laroche F, Perrot S, Medkour T, et al. Quality of life and impact of pain in women treated with aromatase inhibitors for breast cancer: A multicenter cohort study. *PLoS One*. 2017;12(11):e0187165.

12 Cold-Evoked Symptoms After Chemotherapy

Lise Ventzel and Nanna Brix Finnerup

A 56-year-old man had surgery for colorectal cancer
and then adjuvant chemotherapy with oxaliplatin.
After the second cycle, he reported pain in the
hands and feet when touching something cold, and
pricking in the mouth and throat when drinking
something cold, lasting 7 days. After the third cycle,
he reported tingling in both feet and the last dose
of oxaliplatin was reduced. During the next months,
cold dysesthesia and pain in the hands decreased
while the symptoms in the feet progressed. One year
after surgery, he describes unpleasant tingling when
walking on a cold surface, numbness, cotton ball
sensation under the feet, and instability with walking,
particularly at night. He was treated with codeine
but states that the drug has no effect. He has several
questions. Are his symptoms a sign of relapse? Will
they continue to progress? Will he ever get rid of
them? Why does codeine does not work?

What do you do now?

This patient treated for colorectal cancer presents with chronic sensory symptoms that started concomitantly with chemotherapy with oxaliplatin and progressed although chemotherapy was stopped. He describes unpleasant tingling when walking on a cold surface (cold dysesthesia), numbness, cotton ball sensation (paresthesia), and postural instability with falls particularly at night. The latter suggests proprioceptive ataxia because proprioceptive deficits are enhanced by the lack of visual feedback (e.g., at night). In this patient with neuropathic symptoms at the feet in the context of chemotherapy with oxaliplatin, the diagnosis of chemotherapy-induced neuropathy is possible.

To confirm the diagnosis, clinical examination is sufficient at this step. This patient has fine tactile deficit at the feet, loss of sense of movement of the toes, vibration deficit, and Romberg ataxia (he tends to fall when standing with his eyes shut) but no thermoalgesic, motor deficit, or reflex abnormalities. This indicates tactile and proprioceptive deficits and goes well with the fact that he has difficulty walking in the dark, and feels cotton ball sensation under the feet. His clinical presentation is compatible with the diagnosis of sensory neuropathy affecting predominantly large myelinated fibers, akin to other chemotherapy-induced neuropathies (Table 12.1). If you have doubts (e.g., if the clinical examination is normal despite sensory symptoms), you may require complementary investigations in specialized settings (particularly electromyography with nerve conduction study).

To ascertain the presence of neuropathic pain, you might be tempted to use a screening questionnaire (see Chapter 1), but this patient does not report pain: he complains of cold-evoked tingling. This is described by the patient as unpleasant but not painful. Thus, screening questionnaires, which have been validated for painful patients, are not relevant here. Importantly, two-thirds of patients with chemotherapy-induced neuropathy do not suffer from pain but, rather, from paresthesia or dysesthesia (only one-third have pain). The latter refer to positive sensations such as numbness, tingling, itch, pins and needles, or cotton ball sensation (as mentioned previously, these symptoms may be associated with proprioceptive deficits), but only dysesthesia is felt as really unpleasant. For these patients, pain treatments are not useful. This is probably why most trials of chemotherapy-induced neuropathies with agents generally effective for neuropathic pain

TABLE 12.1 **Chemotherapy-Induced Neuropathies**

Chemotherapies most commonly responsible for neuropathies	Platins (cisplatin, oxaliplatin, carboplatin) Taxanes (taxotere, taxol) Bortezomid Vinca alkaloids (vinctistine, vinblastine)
Characteristics of acute neuropathy	Specific to oxaliplatin (up to 90% acute symptoms after infusion, subsiding partially after each cycle) Symptoms: tingling, cold allodynia, and dysesthesia in hands, feet, and orofacial area Sometimes pharyngolaryngeal dysesthesia (a feeling that breathing is difficult)
Characteristics of chronic neuropathy	Dose dependent and correlated with cumulative doses (one-third of patients) Sensory loss, paraesthesia, dysesthesia, sometimes pain (one-third of cases) in a typical "glove-and-stocking-like" distribution mainly at the feet
How to diagnose and assess chronic neuropathy	Diagnosis mainly clinical. In painful patients, screening questionnaires (DN4, LANSS, PainDETECT) (see Chapter 1) may differentiate neuropathic from other types of pain. As for other sensory neuropathies, examination should focus on the search for sensory deficits in a typical "glove-and-stocking" distribution at the hands or feet with regard to proprioceptive or fine tactile deficits (vibration, sense of movement, fine tactile discrimination), suggestive of large fiber dysfunction, or to thermoalgesic deficits (warm, cold, pinprick), suggesting small fiber dysfunction (see also Chapter 1). Reflex abnormalities are rare. Complementary examinations to confirm sensory neuropathy (e.g., EMG, laser evoked potentials, skin punch biopsy) required if there are atypical symptoms/signs or normal examination. Specific questionnaires (EORTC-CIPN20, CIPN15, FACT/GOG-Ntx) may assess impact on quality of life.

(continued)

TABLE 12.1 **Continued**

Therapeutic management of neuropathic pain and neuropathic symptoms	Do not use drugs if patient only reports paresthesia.
	Consider physical therapy in case of severe proprioceptive deficits or ataxia.
	For neuropathic pain, use drugs recommended by scientific societies as first or second line (see Chapter 2 for details). Drugs recommended as first line include gabapentin (1200–3600 mg per day in 3 divided doses), pregabalin (150–600 mg per day in 2 or 3 divided doses), duloxetine (30 mg the first week during meal and then 60 mg per day during meal, caution because of several drug drug interactions), amitriptyline or other tricyclic antidepressants (10–75 mg once daily in the evening, reduce the dose in older patients). Second line drugs include topical agents to cover the pain area (lidocaine plasters one to three plasters for 12 hours per day; high-concentration capsaicin patches one to four patches every 3 months). Sustained-release tramadol may also be considered second line (200–400 mg per day) (avoid in combination with high doses antidepressants).
	Do *not* use strong opioids as first line (this is a third-line treatment for neuropathic pain) even if the pain is severe because the World Health Organization analgesic bladder is irrelevant here (chemotherapy-induced neuropathy is a sequelae of cancer and not a sign of progressive cancer).

CIPN15, Chemotherapy-Induced Peripheral Neuropathy 15-item scale; DN4, Douleur Neuropathique 4 questionnaire; EMA, European Medicines Agency; EMG, electromyography; EORTC-CIPN20, European Organization for Research and Treatment of Cancer Quality of Life Questionnaire—Chemotherapy-Induced Peripheral Neuropathy 20-item scale; FACT/GOG-Ntx; Functional Assessment of Cancer Therapy/Gynecologic Oncology Group–Neurotoxicity; FDA, U.S. Food and Drug Administration; LANSS, Leeds Assessment of Neuropathic Symptoms and Signs.

(gabapentin, lidocaine plasters, etc.) were negative: Patients enrolled in these trials had mainly paresthesia or dysesthesia. The only exception concerns duloxetine, which has been found to be effective in a trial of painful chemotherapy-induced neuropathy: in this trial, patients had moderate to severe pain at inclusion.

You should now reassure the patient and respond to his questions. His symptoms are not a sign of relapse but are a sequaelae of his chemotherapy; hence, they should not continue to progress, and their presence does not mean that the cancer will progress. Codeine cannot be of any benefit for his symptoms because it is not appropriate for neuropathic pain, and he has no pain. So he has to progressively taper off the treatment. You should also explain to him that his disability (falls and sensation of cotton balls) will be best managed by proprioceptive therapy by a physiotherapist.

This patient tapered off codeine and started physical therapy focused on proprioception. He now walks better and does not fall anymore. He still feels tingling or numbness, but because he now understands that these symptoms are not related to cancer progression, he copes better with them and his quality of life has improved.

Of note, this patient also reported symptoms during the acute phase of oxaliplatin therapy, consisting mainly of pain of the hands and feet when touching something cold, suggestive of cold allodynia, and of pricking of the mouth and throat when drinking something cold (cold orofacial dysesthesia). Of all chemotherapies, only oxaliplatin causes acute and chronic neuropathies. This case illustrates a common situation—the relief of acute neuropathy after the end of chemotherapy while symptoms in the lower extremities progress despite stopping chemotherapy (the "coasting effect"). However, chronic neuropathy with oxaliplatin may occur without being preceded by acute neuropathy, which makes it difficult for clinicians to know when to reduce or stop the treatment. The patient had been informed of the potential risks of toxicity with oxaliplatin and asked to report acute symptoms. He did not receive specific therapy before oxaliplatin, as no agent has been clearly demonstrated to effectively prevent chemotherapy-induced neuropathy, but the dosages of oxaliplatin were reduced during the fourth cycle to reduce the risk of enhanced neurotoxicity.

- Oxaliplatin used in colorectal cancer causes both acute and chronic neuropathy.
- Chronic oxaliplatin-induced neuropathy is dose dependent and correlated to cumulative dose.
- No agent has been found effective in the prevention of chemotherapy-induced neuropathy.
- Patients with chemotherapy-induced neuropathy reporting paresthesia such as numbness or tingling but not pain should not be treated with analgesics.
- Analgesic therapy for chronic oxaliplatin-induced painful neuropathy should not start with opioids and is similar to that for other peripheral neuropathic pain conditions.

Further Reading

Bennedsgaard K, Ventzel L, Themistocleous AC, et al. Long-term symptoms of polyneuropathy in breast and colorectal cancer patients treated with and without adjuvant chemotherapy. *Cancer Med*. 2020;9(14):5114–5123.

Bonhof CS, van de Poll-Franse LV, Vissers PAJ, et al. Anxiety and depression mediate the association between chemotherapy-induced peripheral neuropathy and fatigue: Results from the population-based PROFILES registry. *Psychooncology*. 2019;28(9):1926–1933.

Finnerup NB, Attal N, Haroutounian S, et al. Pharmacotherapy for neuropathic pain in adults: A systematic review and meta-analysis. *Lancet Neurol*. 2015;14(2):162–173.

Loprinzi CL, Lacchetti C, Bleeker J, et al. Prevention and management of chemotherapy-induced peripheral neuropathy in survivors of adult cancers: ASCO guideline update. *J Clin Oncol*. 2020;38(28):3325–3348.

Staff NP, Grisold A, Grisold W, et al. Chemotherapy-induced peripheral neuropathy: A current review. *Ann Neurol*. 2017;81(6):772–781.

13 Cervicobrachial Pain and Cancer

Nadine Attal and Didier Bouhassira

A 67-year-old man operated on for lung cancer 2 years ago presents with a unique bone metastasis at the cervical level, for which immunotherapy and surgery are being considered by his oncologist team. He reports moderate burning pain in the inner part of the right arm, forearm, and hand (rated 5 out of 10 on a 0–10 numerical pain scale), and severe pain paroxysms (at least twenty times a day, rated 9 out of 10) described as electric shocks, associated with tingling and pins and needles. He also complains of neck pain, described as aching, heavy, dull, and increased by movements. Examination shows absent ulnar tendon reflexes on the right arm, sensory deficit in the painful upper limb and pyramidal syndrome (spasticity, hyperreflexia, Babinski sign) on the left leg. He receives sustained-release morphine (60 mg per day), with good efficacy on his neck pain but not on his arm pain.

What do you do now?

This man has cervical and arm pain in the context of an unique bone metastasis due to lung cancer. You should first ask him whether his pain is similar in these two body areas and, if not, ask him to describe each pain type. You may use screening questionnaires; the LANSS and DN4 (see Chapter 1) are the most suitable to distinguish between neuropathic and nonneuropathic pain types in the cancer setting.

The patient reports two distinct pain areas. His arm pain is described as burning, with innumerable pain paroxysms (>30 per day) described as electric shocks; it is associated with tingling and pins and needles. It covers the inner part of the right arm, forearm, and hand, which suggests radicular pain (C8 dermatoma). At examination, ulnar tendon reflexes are absent, and there is sensory deficit in the inner part of the right hand, arm, and shoulder. The score on the DN4 questionnaire is 7/10, suggesting neuropathic pain. In contrast, neck pain is described as aching, heavy, dull, and increased by neck movements, and there is no sensory deficit, which is not in favor of neuropathic pain. The rest of the examination discloses moderate spasticity, hyperreflexia, and Babinski sign on the left leg, which indicate pyramidal tract lesion.

Thus, this man with cervical metastasis suffers from chronic cervical pain, which is probably directly related to his metastasis (nociceptive pain), and radicular pain. Furthermore, he has pyramidal tract dysfunction at the lower limb. This suggests that his vertebral cervical lesion is responsible for compressive radiculopathy and myelopathy (metastatic epiduritis).

This man has pain paroxyms in the arm despite sustained-released morphine. Should you consider oromucosal fentanyl? These opioid agonists are indicated for breakthrough pain in cancer adult patients who are receiving around-the-clock opioid therapy (at least 60 mg of oral morphine per day) for their underlying persistent cancer pain. However, although this patient reports pain paroxysms, the latter are innumerable, described specifically as electric shocks; associated with burning, tingling, and pins and needles; and felt in an area of sensory deficit. These pain paroxysms correspond to neuropathic symptoms and resemble those observed in other neuropathic conditions, particularly trigeminal neuralgia (in which transmucosal fentanyl is not an option). Their mechanisms are probably distinct from those of most cases of breakthrough pains, which are mainly related to specific neurochemical mechanisms after bone injury. In this context, rather

TABLE 13.1 **Main Neuropathic Pain Syndromes in Patients with Cancer**

Cancer or Its Treatment	Type of Nerve Lesions	Mechanisms or Causes
Cancer		
Solid tumors	Peripheral nerve lesions	Paraspinal/retroperitoneal mass Chest wall mass Other soft tissue or bony tumor Polyneuropathy
	Radiculopathy or cauda equina syndrome	Vertebral lesion Leptomeningeal metastasis Other intraspinal neoplasms
	Plexopathy	Cervical, brachial, lumbosacral
	Cranial neuropathy	Base of skull tumors Leptomeningeal metastases Other soft tissue or bony cranial tumors
	Central nervous system lesion	Myelopathy Intracerebral lesion
Hematologic malignancy	Peripheral neuropathies	Neuropathy due to paraproteins Amyloidosis
	Plexopathy	Tumor invasion Node enlargement compression (lymphomas)
	Central nervous system lesion	Myelopathy Intracerebral lesion
Cancer treatment		
Radiotherapy	Plexopathy	Radiation plexopathy
	Peripheral nerve lesions	Radiation injury to nerves
Chemotherapy	Peripheral neuropathies	Oxaliplatin, cisplatin, bortezomid, taxane, paclixatel, vinka alcaloids
Surgery	Peripheral nerve lesions	Post-mastectomy pain Post-thoracotomy pain Other

Adapted and modified from Caraceni and Shkodra (2019).

than introducing oromucosal fentanyl, it is advisable to introduce an antineuropathic drug. You may therefore continue oral morphine without increasing dosages and add pregabalin starting with 75 mg in the evening and then titrating by steps of 75 mg every 2 or 3 days up to efficacy or side effects for up to 600 mg per day. Pregabalin may have additive effects with morphine and has no drug–drug interaction. It may alleviate both burning and paroxysmal pains. This man received oral pregabalin titrated to 450 mg per day, which reduced the number of pain paroxysms to only one or two per day and their intensity by 50%.

Inadequate assessment of neuropathic pain in cancer may have a negative impact on treatment outcomes. Yet neuropathic pain affects up to 40% of cancer patients. It is associated with increased pain intensity, analgesic consumption, and decreased quality of life. Most neuropathic pain mechanisms in cancer patients are related to lesions of nervous tissue due to solid tumors or hematologic malignancies, but pain types are often mixed, combining neuropathic and nociceptive mechanisms. Other mechanisms for neuropathic pain are caused by cancer treatments such as surgery, radiotherapy, or chemotherapy (Table 13.1).

KEY POINTS TO REMEMBER

- Up to 40% of patients with cancer suffer from neuropathic pain.
- Screening questionnaires may help differentiate predominantly neuropathic from predominantly nociceptive pain in cancer patients.
- The management of neuropathic cancer pain is difficult, but international recommendations for neuropathic pain management encompass neuropathic cancer pain, and the main specificity compared to non-cancer pain is the fact that pain may occur in a palliative context.
- Although transmucosal fentanyl is indicated for breakthrough pain in the context of cancer in patients receiving stable opioid therapy, other therapeutic options such as antineuropathic agents are more relevant for electric shock like pain even in patients with cancer, as the latter correspond mainly to neuropathic symptoms.

Further Reading

Bennett MI, Rayment C, Hjermstad M, Aass N, Caraceni A, Kaasa S. Prevalence and aetiology of neuropathic pain in cancer patients: A systematic review. *Pain.* 2012;153(2):359–365.

Caraceni A, Shkodra M. Cancer pain assessment and classification. *Cancers.* 2019;11(4):510.

Gouveia AG, Chan DCW, Hoskin PJ, et al. Advances in radiotherapy in bone metastases in the context of new target therapies and ablative alternatives: A critical review. *Radiother Oncol.* 2021;163:55–67.

Moisset X, Bouhassira D. Avez Couturier J, et al. Pharmacological and non-pharmacological treatments for neuropathic pain: Systematic review and French recommendations. *Rev Neurol.* 2020;176(5):325–352.

Mulvey MR, Boland EG, Bouhassira D, et al. Neuropathic pain in cancer: Systematic review, performance of screening tools and analysis of symptom profiles. *Br J Anaesth.* 2017;119(4):765–774.

14 My Body Is Boiling

Nadine Attal, Didier Bouhassira, and Andrea Truini

A 65-year-old woman developed pain 4 years ago
initially involving the toes and feet and described as
hot/burning and electric shocks. She has no significant
medical history except for hypertension and a major
depressive episode 15 years ago. Three years ago,
her pain started to extend to the lower limbs, then
upper limbs. She now reports severe continuous
pain "all over the body" (rated 7 out of 10 on a 0–10
numeric rating scale). She also complains of fatigue,
insomnia, micturition problems, and feels anxious
and stressed (her husband died 2 years ago from
cancer). She consulted a neurologist because of
memory and attention loss; she is afraid of having
Alzheimer disease like her mother. The neurologist
performed a skin punch biopsy at the ankle, which
showed a reduction of intraepidermal nerve fibers.
Complementary biological investigations to explore
potential causes for sensory neuropathy were normal.

What do you do now?

This woman reports chronic widespread pain and multiple associated symptoms. However, her pain was not widespread when it initially started. Rather, it was restricted to the feet bilaterally and described as typically neuropathic (burning and electric shocks). This is compatible with a sensory neuropathy. Skin punch biopsy at the ankle (Chapter 38) showed a reduction of intraepidermal nerve fibers. This suggests small fiber neuropathy (a selective or predominant impairment of nociceptive fibers characterized by sensory deficits and generally neuropathic pain in a bilateral and symmetric topographical distribution in distal parts of the limbs) (see Chapter 38).

Now this woman's widespread pain is constant; associated with multiple symptoms, including fatigue, insomnia, micturition problems, and anxiety; and has a major impact on her ability to concentrate. Such clinical presentation is compatible with fibromyalgia.

The best therapeutic strategy is multimodal, in keeping with updated recommendations for fibromyalgia. Psychoeducation is essential. You have to explain to her the mechanisms of pain with simple words in order to reassure her. You might state, for example, that although her pain was perhaps initially related to a neuropathy, the spread of pain to the whole body was probably related to her stress. You should also tell her that the fact that no cause was found for her neuropathy is not a concern because pain may evolve independently of the cause and that her therapeutic management should target her symptoms and not the cause of her pain (moreover, even if there is a curable cause, such as diabetes, the treatment of pain is often mandatory). You may propose drug therapy, and we advise you to consider duloxetine 30 mg daily for 7 days during meal and then 60 mg once daily (U.S. Food and Drug Administration approved for chronic musculoskeletal pain). This should be best associated with physical reconditioning and, if possible, cognitive–behavior therapy with a psychologist.

This woman received cognitive therapy, physical therapy, and duloxetine 60 mg per day. Her pain is still present but more limited (rated as 5 or 6/10), and her coping abilities have improved.

The revised American College of Rheumatology diagnostic criteria (2016) for fibromyalgia include diffuse widespread pain, defined as pain in at least four of five body regions (excluding chest, jaw, and abdomen); symptoms for at least 3 months; and several associated symptoms, including those reported by this woman (e.g., fatigue, sleep disorders, mood disorders, and cognitive complaints). Of note, screening neuropathic pain questionnaires are not adapted for widespread pain because they were validated for patients with focal pain. Other questionnaires, such as the six-item Fibromyalgia Rapid Screening Tool (FiRST), may help differentiate fibromyalgia from diffuse osteoarthritis or arthritis (Box 14.1). This woman scores 6/6 on the FiRST, which is in favor of fibromyalgia.

Fibromyalgia is considered as nociplastic pain ("pain that arises from altered nociception despite no clear evidence of actual tissue damage causing the pain") by opposition to neuropathic pain and nociceptive/inflammatory pains (see Chapter 1). It may classically develop in the context of rheumatological diseases, such as chronic arthritis or spondylosis, but also in relation with stress, sleep disorders, past traumatic events, or any focal painful injury (e.g., whiplash, sciatica, and low back pain).

This woman's widespread pain and her multiple symptoms were associated with small fiber neuropathy. Several recent studies have outlined the frequent association between small fiber neuropathy and fibromyalgia. Because small fibers mediate multiple autonomic functions (including sudomotor, thermoregulatory, cardiovascular, gastrointestinal, and

BOX 14.1 **Fibromyalgia Rapid Screening Tool**		
	Yes	No
I have pain all over my body.		
My pain is accompanied by a continuous and very unpleasant general fatigue.		
My pain feels like burns, electric shocks, or cramps.		
My pain is accompanied by other unusual sensations throughout my body, such as pins and needles, tingling, or numbness.		
My pain is accompanied by other health problems, such as digestive problems, urinary problems, headaches, or restless legs.		
My pain has a significant impact on my life, particularly on my sleep and my ability to concentrate, making me feel slower generally.		

This scale has been validated in patients with widespread pain. A score of 5/6 strongly suggests fibromyalgia with 90.5% sensitivity and 86% specificity.
Adapted from Perrot et al. (2010).

urogenital functions), it cannot be excluded that small fiber neuropathy might account for almost all this woman's symptoms, keeping in mind that cognitive and affective disorders might be the consequence of pain and sleep disorders. Another possibility is that the spread of pain from focal areas to her whole body was related to central mechanisms (i.e., central sensitization and/or dysfunction of central pain modulatory systems). In all cases, the role of chronic stress in this woman should not be neglected and might even have been a trigger for her initial impairment of small nociceptive fibers.

KEY POINTS TO REMEMBER

- Fibromyalgia may be associated with painful (small fiber) neuropathy, but it is unclear whether the neuropathy is a trigger or may cause the pain and associated symptoms in fibromyalgia syndrome.
- Therapeutic management should be based on the clinical phenotype. For fibromyalgia syndrome, recommendations include mainly therapeutic education, physical reconditioning, and cognitive–behavior therapy.

Further Reading

Grayston R, Czanner G, Elhadd K, et al. A systematic review and meta-analysis of the prevalence of small fiber pathology in fibromyalgia: Implications for a new paradigm in fibromyalgia etiopathogenesis. *Semin Arthritis Rheum.* 2019;48(5):933–940.

Macfarlane GJ, Kronisch C, Atzeni F, et al. EULAR recommendations for management of fibromyalgia. *Ann Rheum Dis.* 2017;76(12):e54.

Nicholas M, Vlaeyen JWS, Rief W, et al. IASP Taskforce for the Classification of Chronic Pain. The IASP classification of chronic pain for ICD-11: chronic primary pain. *Pain.* 2019;160(1):28–37.

Perrot S, Bouhassira D, Fermanian J; CEDR (Cercle d'Etude de la Douleur en Rhumatologie). Development and validation of the Fibromyalgia Rapid Screening Tool (FiRST). *Pain.* 2010;150(2):250–256.

15 Pain and COVID-19

Daniel Ciampi de Andrade

A 59-year-old woman complains of persistent pain
in the four limbs that started after intensive care
unit discharge due to COVID-19 (delta variant).
Before ICU, she had received one injection of
COVID-19 vaccine. She developed severe respiratory
symptoms, for which she underwent mechanical
ventilation for 3 weeks. After her ventilatory function
improved, intensive care physicians noticed that
she had difficulty weaning from the ventilator and
presented flaccid weakness of the four limbs. Nerve
conduction studies and cerebrospinal fluid analysis
fulfilled criteria for Guillain–Barré syndrome. CSF
polymerase chain reaction tests for infectious agents
were negative except for COVID-19. She received
intravenous human immunoglobulin and regained
motor function within weeks. As she woke up from
sedation, she complained of tingling, electric shock-
like and burning pain over her feet and fingers. She
lost 20 pounds since COVID-19 and reports extreme
fatigue and sleep disorders. She also has renal
insufficiency (creatinine clearance is 38 mg/ml).

What do you do now?

This woman suffers from persistent pain involving the four limbs following Guillain Barré syndrome (GBS) in the context of COVID-19 infection.

This woman's pain has neuropathic characteristics (electric shocks and burning) and persists despite over-the-counter analgesics weeks after discharge from hospital. Although GBS is primarily paralytic and demyelinating (affecting the myelin sheath), it also affects small fibers (nociceptive and autonomic), thus contributing to her persisting neuropathic pain, and the prolonged ICU stay might also be a trigger for her persisting pain.

The first-line management of neuropathic pain for this patient should follow international guidelines for peripheral neuropathic pain (see Chapter 2). You may consider starting with pregabalin, gabapentin, duloxetine, or tricyclic antidepressants. This woman lost weight since COVID-19 and has sleep disorders. She has renal insufficiency, which is a contraindication to gabapentinoids (at least at this point; it is possible that her renal insufficiency will progressively recover because it may be partially functional). Hence, it is advised to use a tricyclic antidepressant, albeit at low dosages, which may be effective for neuropathic pain, contribute to increase her weight, and improve her sleep. You may start with amitriptyline (in drops) 10 mg every evening (its use in the morning should be avoided because of the risk of somnolence) and then increase by steps of 10 mg every 4–7 days based on efficacy and side effects. Common side effects include somnolence, confusion, dry mouth, constipation, postural hypotension, and weight gain. Electrocardiography is recommended at baseline to assess the QT interval. This patient's electrocardiogram was normal. This woman started with amitriptyline 10 mg every evening and now receives amitriptyline 40 mg once daily in the evening with acceptable tolerability (except for mild somnolence and dry mouth) and good efficacy on her residual pain.

GBS is an autoimmune disorder of peripheral nerves with an acute onset. The prevalence of GBS is estimated to be 15 in 100,000 COVID-19 patients, but it remains to be determined whether COVID-19 infection confers a higher than expected prevalence of GBS compared to other viral diseases (Table 15.1). Diagnosis is based on the presence of progressive muscle weakness in more than one limb in a mainly symmetric distribution (areflexia), but sensory symptoms and dysautonomia are also important. CSF shows normal or reduced (<50) leukocytes and often raised protein levels. Nerve conduction tests may be subsequently altered (generally after 1 week). Recovery usually takes months.

Another type of pain following severe COVID-19 in the ICU is post-ICU neuromuscular disorder (50–100% of ICU patients). It encompasses critical-illness polyneuropathy or myopathy and acute necrotizing myopathy. It is caused by energy failure and microvasculature damage of peripheral nerves and muscles. Risk factors include immobilization, sepsis,

TABLE 15.1 **Neuropathic Pain After COVID-19 and Other Viral Infections**

Virus Responsible for Neurological Lesions That May Induce Neuropathic Pain	Neurological Lesions
Herpes zoster	Lesion of sensory ganglia (responsible for postherpetic neuralgia) Myelitis
Human immunodeficiency virus	Painful sensory polyneuropathy Myelitis
Enteroviruses	Myelitis
Poliovirus	Post-polio syndrome
HTLV1	Myelitis
Zika	Guillain–Barré syndrome
Chikungunja	Myelitis
Other virusesa	Guillain–Barré syndrome
COVID-19	Guillain–Barré syndrome Post ICU polyneuropathy Myelitisb Strokeb

aFor example, Epstein–Barr virus, cytomegalovirus, influenza A, coronaviruses, and hepatitis.

bAlthough, myelitis and stroke may cause neuropathic pain, the exact prevalence of neuropathic pain due to these neurological lesions after COVID-19 is currently unknown.

ICU, intensive care unit.

Adapted from Attal et al. (2021).

older age, and metabolic factors (hyperosmolality, hemodialysis, and hyperglycemia). The acute clinical presentation is proximal weakness, usually sparing the facial and ocular muscles, and difficulty weaning from mechanical ventilation. Specific treatments include early mobilization and minimization of sedation and mechanical ventilation duration. Patients may subsequently report chronic neuropathic pain (critical illness neuropathy) or muscle pain (myopathy). COVID-19 has also (rarely) been reported to induce myelitis, as is the case for other viruses (Table 15.1) and stroke in severe cases, which may also induce neuropathic pain.

Other chronic pains that may develop after moderate to severe COVID-19 infections are not neuropathic and part of long COVID or post-COVID syndrome. These consist of a constellation of symptoms, including headache or widespread pain, fatigue, respiratory or cardiovascular problems, and sleep disorders. These symptoms, which share similarities with other post-infectious disorders, might result from residual damage from acute infection, persistent immune activation, psychological factors, or unmasking of prior comorbidities.

KEY POINTS TO REMEMBER

- Guillain–Barré syndrome has been reported to occur after COVID-19 and may induce neuropathic pain through an impairment of small nociceptives fibers.
- Other causes of pain after COVID-19 are not necessarily neuropathic and mainly include post-ICU neuromuscular disorders for severe cases and long COVID syndrome.

Further Reading

Al-Aly Z, Xie Y, Bowe B. High-dimensional characterization of post-acute sequelae of COVID-19. *Nature*. 2021;594(7862):259–264.

Attal N, Martinez V, Bouhassira D. Potential for increased prevalence of neuropathic pain after the COVID-19 pandemic. *Pain Rep*. 2021;6(1):e884.

Greene-Chandos D, Torbey M. Critical care of neuromuscular disorders. *Continuum*. 2018;24(6):1753–1775.

Martinez V, Fletcher D, Martin F, et al. Small fibre impairment predicts neuropathic pain in Guillain–Barré syndrome. *Pain*. 2010;151(1):53–60.

Palaiodimou L, Stefanou MI, Katsanos AH, et al. Prevalence, clinical characteristics and outcomes of Guillain–Barré syndrome spectrum associated with COVID-19: A systematic review and meta-analysis. *Eur J Neurol.* 2021;28(10):3517–3529.

Soares FHC, Kubota GT, Fernandes AM, et al.; Pain in the Pandemic Initiative Collaborators. Prevalence and characteristics of new-onset pain in COVID-19 survivors, a controlled study. *Eur J Pain.* 2021;25(6):1342–1354.

Stoian A, Bălașa R, Grigorescu BL, et al. Guillain–Barré syndrome associated with COVID-19: A close relationship or just a coincidence? [Review]. *Exp Ther Med.* 2021;22(3):916.

16 Perineal Pain

Nadine Attal and Didier Bouhassira

A 39-year-old man consults for a right perineal pain
that started 2 years ago. He has no notable past
medical history. Pain started after intensive horseback
riding and cycling during vacations (he is an
excellent horse rider and amateur cyclist). It is rated
at 8 on a 0–10 numerical rating scale and involves
the genital organs (scrotal skin). Pain is described
as burning and stabbing, increased by sitting,
sensitive to clothes and underwear, and alleviated by
standing; it is not present at night. He admits having
occasional impotence problems. Urinalysis with
culture, semen analysis, and pelvic and transrectal
prostatic ultrasounds are normal. Magnetic resonance
imaging (MRI) of the abdominal and pelvic area is
normal. Antibiotics, antimycotics, paracetamol, and
nonsteroidal anti-inflammatory agents are ineffective.

What do you do now?

This man reports chronic perineal pain involving the genitals. The description of his pain is crucial because the clinical examination may be difficult or poor. He describes spontaneous burning and stabbing pain, and pain is increased by underwear, which probably refers to tactile allodynia. These are neuropathic characteristics. The score on the PainDETECT screening questionnaire (see Chapters 1 and 4) is 23, which strongly suggests neuropathic pain (cutoff value ≥ 19).

Thus, this man probably suffers from perineal neuropathic pain, which tends to rule out nonneuropathic causes of chronic perineal pains in men such as chronic prostatitis. This is confirmed here by normal complementary examinations including pelvic MRI, which excludes pelvic tumor. Pain started after intensive horseback riding and cycling during vacations. It involves the right genitals only, is increased by sitting, and is alleviated by standing. This is characteristic of pudendal neuralgia.

This patient was initially treated with pregabalin but stopped the drug because of side effects. He does not wish to receive other oral drug therapy,

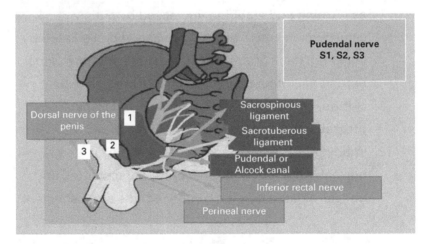

FIGURE 16.1 The pudendal nerve is one of the main causes of pelviperineal pain. It emerges from the S2, S3, and S4 roots ventral rami of the sacral plexus (1), then passes under the piriformis muscle, leaves the pelvis through the lower part of the greater sciatic foramen, and crosses the sacrospinous and sacrotuberous ligament (close to its insertion to the ischial spine) (2). Then, after re-entering the pelvis, it courses through the pudendal canal (Alcock canal—a structure formed by the fascia of the obturator internus muscle) (3). Inside the pudendal canal, the nerve divides into branches, giving off the inferior rectal nerve and then the perineal nerve, before continuing as the dorsal nerve of the penis or clitoris.

TABLE 16.1 Main Clinical Characteristics and Treatment of Pudendal Neuralgia

Pain characteristics	Described as neuropathic: burning/hot, shooting, allodynia to brush Screening questionnaires helpful (DN4, PainDETECT, LANSS) (Chapter 1)
Pain territory	Genitals, perineum, and anorectal region Unilateral
Context	Entrapment: pregnancy, congenital, surgery, radiotherapy, horse riding, biking Pelvic tumor, sacral nerve root involvement or stretch neuropathy of the pudendal nerve (after delivery in women)
Clinical and complementary investigations	Clinical examination sometimes normal because of the frequent overlapping of nerve territories or showing sensory deficit Rectal or vaginal examination: tenderness on palpation of the ischial spine Electromyography of the perineal floor, bulbocavernosus reflex: differentiates pudendal entrapment neuropathy from other pudendal pains Pelvic MRI: rules out compressive causes due to tumor
Associated symptoms	Urinary frequency Erectile dysfunction Pain after sexual intercourse
Factors improving or increasing the pain	Pain increased by sitting or defecation Pain alleviated by standing or at night
Management	Similar to that of neuropathic pain Pudendal nerve blockade (local anesthetics, corticosteroids) may induce long-term effects Surgical transgluteal decompression and transposition of the nerve, spinal cord stimulation, and motor cortex rTMS for refractory cases

rTMS, repetitive transcranial magnetic stimulation.

and topical therapy with 5% lidocaine plasters was insufficient. You may refer him for pudendal nerve blocks with local anesthetics or corticosteroids in specialist settings. These blocks sometimes have long-term efficacy. This patient underwent two pudendal nerve blocks within 6 months, with more than 70% sustained pain relief. He was advised to reduce biking and horseback riding and to envisage other sports, and he ultimately decided to practice swimming.

Pudendal neuralgia is a major cause of chronic perineal neuropathic pain and is most commonly due to pudendal nerve entrapment in the Alcock canal, often caused by excessive cycling or horseback riding (Table 16.1; Figure 16.1). Management is difficult, and there are no international guidelines or good quality studies. Because it is a peripheral neuropathic pain, pharmacological management including pregabalin (150–600 mg per day), gabapentin (1200–3600 mg per day), antidepressants (amitriptyline 10–75 mg once daily, duloxetine 60–120 mg once daily), topical agents such as 5% lidocaine patches or even capsaicin high-concentration patches (provided that the pain involves only a cutaneous territory), but also transcutaneous electrical nerve stimulation may be appropriate.

Other lesions of nerves or nerve roots may cause perineal neuropathic pain. These include the gluteal nerve (pain then involves mainly the gluteal or anal region, entrapment or compression being the most prevalent), the hypogastric/ilioinguinal nerve (pain affects mainly the inguinal region and generally occurs after inguinal hernia repair), or the thoracolumbar root (the latter may cause pelvic pain through autonomic impairment but pain is generally more diffuse and bilateral).

KEY POINTS TO REMEMBER

- Pudendal nerve entrapment is the most common cause of pudendal neuralgia.
- Pudendal neuralgia corresponds to a peripheral neuropathic pain and as such may necessitate similar antineuropathic drugs as other neuropathic pains.
- Pudendal nerve blocks may have a diagnostic value and may sometimes induce long-term benefit in this context.

Further Reading

Buffenoir K, Rioult B, Hamel O, et al. Spinal cord stimulation of the conus medullaris for refractory pudendal neuralgia: A prospective study of 27 consecutive cases. *Neurourol Urodyn*. 2015;34(2):177–182.

Labat JJ, Riant T, Lassaux A, et al. Adding corticosteroids to the pudendal nerve block for pudendal neuralgia: A randomised, double-blind, controlled trial. *BJOG*. 2017;124(2):251–260.

Labat JJ, Riant T, Robert R, et al. Diagnostic criteria for pudendal neuralgia by pudendal nerve entrapment (Nantes criteria). *Neurourol Urodyn*. 2008;27(4):306–310.

Robert R, Labat JJ, Bensignor M, et al. Decompression and transposition of the pudendal nerve in pudendal neuralgia: A randomized controlled trial and long-term evaluation. *Eur Urol*. 2005;47(3):403–408.

17 Burning Mouth

Nadine Attal and Didier Bouhassira

A 82-year-old woman was a Spanish teacher for 40
years. Since her retirement at the age of 67 years, she
has been suffering from burning pain in the tongue,
dryness of the mouth, and modifications of taste.
Pain is not increased by brushing the teeth or eating.
It is moderately improved by eating but is worse in
the evening, after talking, or when she is stressed.
It is constant during daytime and troublesome for
everyday activities, but does not impair sleep. She
feels very anxious because she is afraid of having
cancer and states that her life is a mess, particularly
since the death of her husband. She has sought
medical advice, and local mycosis was excluded. She
has seen several dentists, who could not find any
teeth problems. Examination of the tongue is normal,
and there is no apparent sensory deficit. Biological
testing is normal. Acetaminophen and codeine are not
beneficial.

What do you do now?

This woman has pain in the tongue. Her pain appeared progressively, has always been restricted to the tongue, and is bilateral. It is described as continuous burning (no other painful symptoms) and associated with dryness of the mouth and modifications of taste. It is not increased by brushing the teeth or eating; on the contrary, it is improved by chewing gum but is worse in the evening or after talking (this woman was formerly a teacher; it is possible that years of talking loud might have been a trigger of her pain). Pain is constant during daytime, except during meals; it does not disturb the sleep, but it has a major impact on daily activities. Common causes of burning mouth were excluded (e.g., candidosis or vitamin B_{12} deficiency, Sjögren syndrome, diabetes, mucosal lesions, or specific dental or tongue problems). This woman's condition is thus compatible with the diagnosis of burning mouth syndrome (BMS), also called glossodynia or stomatodynia, which predominantly affects postmenopausal women.

You should first tell this woman that she has no evidence of cancer and that BMS is a specific chronic pain. We advise you treat her pain with topical clonazepam 1-mg tablet three times daily, sucked for 3 minutes before spitting (3-month prescription). If pain is not relieved enough, you may add duloxetine 30 mg during meals for 1 week and then 60 mg at meals, which may also reduce her anxiety. You may ask for psychiatric advice or psychological counseling. This woman was started with topical clonazepam, but because this decreased her pain by only 20%, duloxetine 60 mg per day was added. She finally reports 50% efficacy with this combination on her burning sensation, which has become tolerable for daily living (Figure 17.2).

BMS is defined as an intraoral burning or dysesthetic sensation, recurring daily for more than 2 hours per day over more than 3 months, without clinically evident causative lesions. Pain affects the tongue bilaterally, especially its tip and anterior two-thirds, less commonly the palate and gingivae, lower lips, and pharynx (Figure 17.1), and it tends to worsen during the day. The onset is spontaneous or associated with triggers such as a dental procedure, spicy or acidic food, or stress. Eating or using chewing gum may alleviate the pain. Other symptoms and signs include dry mouth (xerostomia), modifications of saliva composition, and

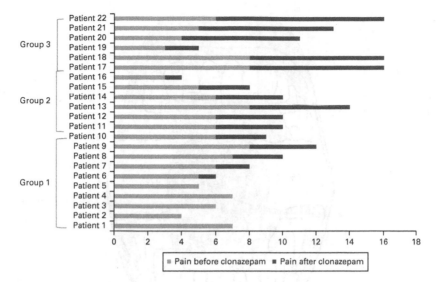

FIGURE 17.1 Effects of local clonazepam (1-mg tablet three times daily, sucked for 3 minutes before spitting) in individual patients with burning mouth syndrome (in a double-blind, placebo-controlled trial). For each patient, the numerical rating scale for pain intensity (NRS) was recorded before treatment and 14 days after the first application. Group 1 corresponded to very successful treatments: The NRS score decreased by 4–7/10. Group 2 corresponded to partially successful treatments: The NRS score decreased by 2 or 3/10. Group 3 corresponded to unsuccessful treatments. These data show that a subset of patients with BMS are relieved by topical clonazepam. They were confirmed in a subsequent double-blind study of peripheral nerve blocks showing that the group of patients with very successful treatment was the one for which peripheral mechanisms were involved in pain relief. Otherwise, BMS may be due to central mechanisms.

Adapted from Gremeau-Richard C, Woda A, Navez ML, Attal N, Bouhassira D, Gagnieu MC, Laluque JF, Picard P, Pionchon P, Tubert S. Topical clonazepam in stomatodynia: a randomised placebo-controlled study. *Pain*. 2004 Mar;108(1-2):51–7.

dysgeusia (altered taste perception). Comorbidities with other orofacial pains, irritable bowel syndrome, widespread pain, and depression are common. The diagnosis is clinical.

Although BMS is not considered as neuropathic (with the lack of an objective nerve lesion), it has many similarities with neuropathic pains in terms

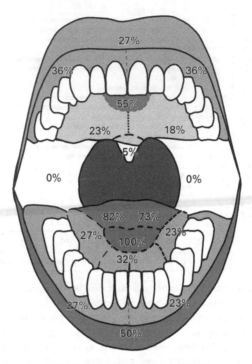

FIGURE 17.2 Most common pain areas in burning mouth syndrome.

of symptoms and mechanisms. Guidelines for neuropathic pain may apply to glossodynia with emphasis on pregabalin, gabapentin, and duloxetine (tricyclics should be avoided because of their risk of mouth dryness). However, there are also specificities. In particular, topical clonazepam (the action of which may be due to effects on $GABA_A$ receptors in the nerve fibers of the oral mucosa) in the form of 1-mg tablets three times daily, sucked for 3 minutes before spitting, has been reported to alleviate pain intensity (compared to placebo) in two-thirds of cases (Figure 17.2). In specialist settings, other topical treatments (salivary substitutes, tongue protectors, and very low doses of capsaicin [0.01%] mixed in xylocaine gel [2%] twice a day) might also be useful. For refractory cases, repetitive transcranial magnetic stimulation of the motor cortex or prefrontal cortex may be proposed (see Chapter 41).

- Primary BMS shares similarities with chronic neuropathic pain.
- Secondary causes, particularly candidosis, should be excluded.
- Treatment is difficult, with weak evidence for efficacy of topical clonazepam.

Further Reading

Grémeau-Richard C, Dubray C, Aublet-Cuvelier B, Ughetto S, Woda A. Effect of lingual nerve block on burning mouth syndrome (stomatodynia): A randomized crossover trial. *Pain.* 2010;149(1):27–32.

Grémeau-Richard C, Woda A, Navez ML, et al. Topical clonazepam in stomatodynia: A randomised placebo-controlled study. *Pain.* 2004;108(1–2):51–57.

Jääskeläinen SK, Woda A. Burning mouth syndrome. *Cephalalgia.* 2017;37(7):627–647.

Nicholas M, Vlaeyen JWS, Rief W, et al; IASP Taskforce for the Classification of Chronic Pain. The IASP classification of chronic pain for ICD-11: Chronic primary pain. *Pain.* 2019;160(1):28–37.

Woda A, Tubert-Jeannin S, Bouhassira D, et al. Towards a new taxonomy of idiopathic orofacial pain. *Pain.* 2005;116(3):396–406.

18 Orofacial Pain

Nadine Attal and Didier Bouhassira

A 32-year-old woman suffers from chronic pain covering the left side of the face, including the forehead, cheek, nose, and chin, and extending to the left cervical area and left shoulder. Pain is continuous, described as hot/burning and aching, without pain paroxysms. She states that her pain is so intense that it necessitates immediate-release oral morphine 10-mg tablets, but she never uses more than three or four tablets per day, depending on her pain intensity (she was prescribed morphine by a primary care provider a few weeks ago). She also reports difficulty sleeping, symptoms of stress, and several panic attacks, to such an extent that she is currently unable to resume her work (she is an executive assistant at a large firm). She has recently separated from her boyfriend because he could not tolerate the situation. At interview, she recalls that her pain appeared after left mandibular third molar avulsion (which was extremely difficult and painful despite local anesthetics), although she does not remember the exact date. Clinical examination is normal.

What do you do now?

This woman reports left hemiface pain after upper maxillary third molar avulsion. Her pain involves the entire left hemiface. It does not cover a neuroanatomical area, is only described as burning, and there is no sensory deficit at examination. This rules out typical neuropathic pain. The most suitable diagnosis is persistent idiopathic facial pain (PIFP), formerly called "atypical facial pain."

In this woman, you should gradually taper off oral morphine, which may have had some initial efficacy on her pain in the short term but is not recommended on a long–term basis because it may ultimately contribute to paradoxically enhance her pain and induce tolerance and dependency on long-term use. This may be done by removing 10 mg per week to her therapeutic regimen. Because she has pain and comorbid anxiety with panic attacks, we advise you to introduce extended-release venlafaxine starting with 37.5 mg in the morning and then increasing by steps of 37.5 mg every week for up to 150 mg per day. Venlafaxine is an antidepressant with serotonin and reuptake inhibitory properties, which is officially approved for use in major depressive episode, generalized anxiety, and panic attacks, but has no official approval for pain, although it may relieve neuropathic pain at high dosages (≥150 mg per day). Main side effects include dizziness, somnolence, constipation, dry mouth, nightmares, bleeding problems, sweating, sexual disorders and weight gain, increased blood pressure, and minor electrocardiogram (ECG) abnormalities (increased QT interval) at high dosages (>150 mg per day) (thus, ECG is recommended at high dosages). You should wait for a few weeks before assessing efficacy of the drug. After at least 6 months, if her pain remains significantly relieved and if there is no outstanding psychiatric condition, you may taper off venlafaxine gradually (to avoid withdrawal syndrome).

This woman started extended-release venlafaxine but could not tolerate doses higher than 112.5 mg per day (75 mg in the morning and 37.5 mg in the evening) because of nightmares and night sweating. She consulted a psychologist and started relaxation. After a few months, she states that her orofacial pain is improved by 50% and that she tolerates it better. She now envisages to reorient her career toward caring because she wishes to help other people like herself.

Persistent idiopathic facial pain is a rare chronic facial pain syndrome characterized by persistent facial and/or oral pain, recurring daily for more than 2 hours per day over more than 3 months, in the absence of clinical neurological deficit. Patients are predominantly female, and pain may not cover a neuroanatomical area but may spread to a large area of the craniocervical region. It may be comorbid with chronic widespread

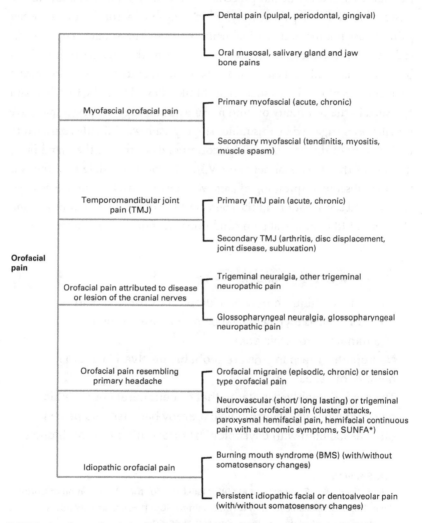

FIGURE 18.1 International classification of orofacial pains.

SUNFA, short-lasting unilateral neuralgiform facial pain attacks with cranial autonomic symptoms.

Adapted and simplified from the International Classification of Orofacial Pain (2020).

pain, irritable bowel syndrome, and psychosocial disorders. Unlike with trigeminal neuralgia, patients have no pain paroxysms (e.g., electric shocks). Although PIFP cannot be considered as neuropathic, there may be a link with neuropathic pain. Many patients with PIFP report traumatic injuries, most commonly dental procedures, in close temporal relation to the onset of their facial pain history, which suggests a continuum between painful post-traumatic trigeminal neuropathy and persistent idiopathic facial pain. Furthermore, mild sensory deficits of the face have sometimes been demonstrated in these patients (based on quantitative sensory testing or neurophysiological tests such as the blink reflex). Here, the fact that pain appeared in the continuity of third molar avulsion suggests that it may have initially been triggered by this minor surgery. Pain was initially restricted to the territory of the left chin, which corresponds to that of the mandibular division of the trigeminal nerve (or V3). The most plausible hypothesis is that the subsequent spreading of pain was due to central functional changes (e.g., central sensitization) in the context of her psychological disorders and life events. Other orofacial pain conditions are indicated in Figure 18.1.

KEY POINTS TO REMEMBER

- There is a continuum between idiopathic orofacial pain (formerly called atypical facial pain) and post-traumatic trigeminal neuropathic pain.
- Neuropathic mechanisms are probably involved in a large number of cases.
- The management is similar to that of peripheral neuropathic pain and includes psychological therapy because this pain is often associated with psychological or psychiatric comorbidities.

Further Reading

Benoliel R, Svensson P, Evers S, et al.; IASP Taskforce for the Classification of Chronic Pain. The IASP classification of chronic pain for ICD-11: Chronic secondary headache or orofacial pain. *Pain*. 2019;160(1):60–68.

Forssell H, Jääskeläinen S, List T, Svensson P, Baad-Hansen L. An update on pathophysiological mechanisms related to idiopathic oro-facial pain conditions with implications for management. *J Oral Rehabil*. 2015;42(4):300–322.

International Classification of Orofacial Pain, 1st edition (ICOP). *Cephalalgia.* 2020;40(2):129–221.

May A, Hoffmann J. Facial pain beyond trigeminal neuralgia. *Curr Opin Neurol.* 2021;34(3):373–377.

Van Deun L, de Witte M, Goessens T, et al. Facial pain: A comprehensive review and proposal for a pragmatic diagnostic approach. *Eur Neurol.* 2020;83(1):5–16.

Woda A, Tubert-Jeannin S, Bouhassira D, et al. Towards a new taxonomy of idiopathic orofacial pain. *Pain.* 2005;116(3):396–406.

Ziegeler C, Schulte LH, May A. Altered trigeminal pain processing on brainstem level in persistent idiopathic facial pain. *Pain.* 2021;162(5):1374–1378.

19 A Lightning in the Face

Andrea Truini and
Gianfranco de Stefano

A 74-year-old otherwise healthy woman comes to medical attention complaining of intense facial pain of recent onset. She describes brief and intense pain attacks, limited to the right side of the face, involving the cheek, upper and lower lips, and the underlying gums. They usually last a fraction of a second, and they sometimes occur in bursts, with many attacks in the span of a few minutes. When asked how she would characterize her pain, she states, "It is like a lighting crossing my face." She notes that the pain is evoked by gentle touch of her upper and lower lips and gums. She also has troubles brushing her teeth, speaking, and chewing, and she has recently lost weight due to poor alimentation. These pain attacks started 2 weeks after a dental procedure. However, her dentist excluded any diseases of the teeth, and her pain is not relieved by over-the-counter painkillers. Her neurological examination is normal.

What do you do now?

This woman complains of paroxysmal electric shock-like pain attacks. Pain is restricted to the right side of the face, involving the cheek, upper and lower lips, and the underlying gum—that is, a cutaneous and mucous territory innervated by the right trigeminal nerve, specifically its second (cheek, upper lips, and underlying gum) and third (lower lips and underlying gum) branches. Pain is evoked by innocuous cutaneous stimulations and maneuvers, which correspond to classical "trigger zones" (also referred to as allodynia). The characteristics of pain, facial distribution, and triggers are typical of trigeminal neuralgia, which is classified as neuropathic pain (Chapter 1). Her neurological examination is unremarkable, contrasting with most other neuropathic conditions (Chapter 1).

You do not need further diagnostic workup to confirm the diagnosis of trigeminal neuralgia. Brain magnetic resonance imaging (MRI; with special sequences for the posterior fossa called constructive interference in steady state [CISS] or fast imaging employing steady-state acquisition) should be conducted to exclude major diseases (multiple sclerosis and tumors of the cerebellopontine angle), even if the neurological examination is normal. In this woman, MRI revealed a superior cerebellar artery impacting the trigeminal nerve root (Figure 19.1). This neurovascular compression with morphological changes of the trigeminal root is a frequent cause of trigeminal

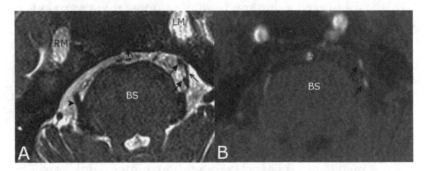

FIGURE 19.1 (A) MRI CISS scans at trigeminal root entry zone level, showing a vascular loop (*bold arrows*) compressing the left trigeminal root (*light arrow*). The left trigeminal root appears distorted by the compression and thinner than the contralateral (*arrowhead*). (B) MRI time-of-flight arterial angiogram (an MRI technique to visualize flow within vessels) taken at the same level as Figure 19.1A, in which the compressing vessel (*arrows*) can be identified as the superior cerebellar artery. BA, basilar artery; BS, brainstem; RM, right Meckel's cave; LM, left Meckel's cave.

neuralgia. If MRI is not possible, trigeminal reflex study (including blink reflex and masseter inhibitory reflex) can be conducted. A normal reflex excludes major disease affecting the trigeminal system.

First-choice treatment for trigeminal neuralgia is different to that of other neuropathic pains and includes the antiepileptics carbamazepine (U.S. Food and Drug Administration and European Medicines Agency label) and oxcarbazepine (off-label) (sodium channel blockers) (Chapter 27). Both have high efficacy: a complete lack of efficacy should put the diagnosis in doubt. Atrioventricular block is the main contraindication, so electrocardiogram (ECG) is recommended before the treatment. Common dose-dependent side effects include central nervous system disturbances (somnolence and dizziness), elevation in liver enzyme, neutropenia, and hyponatremia. With the exception of hyponatremia, they are more common with carbamazepine. Idiosyncratic (unrelated to the dosage) side effects include cutaneous rash and rare cases of Lyell or Stevens–Johnson syndrome.

This woman had a recent normal ECG. You may treat her with oxcarbazepine, starting with 150 mg once or twice a day for the first 3 days, 300 mg twice a day for the next 3 days, and 300 mg three times a day for the next 3 days, which is the therapeutic minimum. You should inform her that somnolence and dizziness are frequent side effects but tend to decrease with the continuation of therapy and to seek medical attention if skin rashes suddenly occur. You should conduct laboratory exams (complete cell blood count, AST, ALT, ALP, GGT, sodium) 2 weeks after reaching therapeutic dosages and then regularly over time (the frequency is not clearly defined). If you prefer to use carbamazepine, then you should opt for immediate-release carbamazepine (sustained-release carbamazepine is more suitable for seizures) and start with 200 mg in the evening for the first 3 days and then increase by 200 mg every 3 days for up to 600 mg TID (maximal dosage 1200 mg TID).

At a return visit 4 weeks later, the woman reporting substantial but not complete pain relief with oxcarbazepine, with a reduction of approximately 60–70% of her pain attacks. Because there was no alteration in her laboratory exams and she only complained of mild dizziness, you may advise her to increase the doses up to the maximum therapeutic dosage of 1800 mg.

How and when should treatment be stopped? The natural history of trigeminal neuralgia comprises periods of spontaneous remission. If your patient achieves a prolonged and complete pain relief with no more attacks, you may slowly reduce medication and eventually suspend it. However, these remission periods are usually transitory, so you should advise the patient to restart the therapy, with the same slow titration, if pain returns. If the patient does not achieve pain relief with the maximum therapeutic dosage or does not tolerate effective doses, you might consider other drugs (off-label; e.g., lamotrigine, gabapentinoids, or botulinum toxin injections in trigger areas in specialized settings) or refer this patient for radiofrequency thermocoagulation of the Gasserian ganglion (may be performed in emergency; the main risk is residual hypoesthesia of the painful area), gamma knife radiosurgery (delayed effect on pain by several months), or microvascular surgical decompression of the posterior fossa (higher risk of morbidity).

KEY POINTS TO REMEMBER

- The diagnosis of trigeminal neuralgia is clinical, and it is characterized by pain limited to the trigeminal territory, occurring in electric shock-like paroxysms and triggered by innocuous cutaneous stimulation or maneuvers.
- In newly diagnosed trigeminal neuralgia, an MRI scan or complete trigeminal reflex testing is mandatory to exclude major neurological diseases.
- First-line therapy is medical and includes carbamazepine or oxcarbazepine. If the occurrence of side effects prevents the patient from reaching the effective dosage, a neurosurgical referral should be considered.

Further Reading

Bendtsen L, Zakrzewska JM, Abbott J, et al. European Academy of Neurology guideline on trigeminal neuralgia. *Eur J Neurol*. 2019;26(6):831–849.

Cruccu G, Di Stefano G, Truini A. Trigeminal neuralgia. *N Engl J Med*. 2020;383(8):754–762.

Di Stefano G, De Stefano G, Leone C, Di Lionardo A, Di Pietro G, Sgro E, Mollica C, Cruccu G, Truini A. Real-world effectiveness and tolerability of carbamazepine and oxcarbazepine in 354 patients with trigeminal neuralgia. *Eur J Pain*. 2021;25(5):1064–1071.

20 Brachial Plexus Avulsion

Daniel Ciampi de Andrade

A 24-year-old man comes to consultation because of hand pain. Pain covers the dorsum of the left hand and has been present since a traumatic brachial plexus avulsion (BPA) while driving a motorcycle 2 years ago. Pain started a few hours after the accident. It is mainly paroxysmal, with intense spontaneous electric shock-like discharges. During the past weeks, he has also experienced a new type of pain, although less severe, over his left shoulder to his left arm and forearm, which is increased by everyday activity and decreased by wearing a sling. This pain is continuous during daytime, described as deep aching. At examination, the patient has complete paralysis of the left arm and extended anesthesia to touch, warm, cold, and pinprick. He was prescribed amitriptyline by his physician, but his pain intensity only decreased by 30% and the treatment induced somnolence and impotence. He seeks other treatment options.

What do you do now?

This young man complains of severe pain of the hand after a traumatic BPA due to a motorcycle accident. He describes his pain as electric shocks involving the left hand, which was totally anesthetic and paralyzed. This is characteristics of neuropathic pain after brachial nerve avulsion (e.g., electric shocks, shooting, and stabbing) (Box 20.1). His pain is restricted to the hand despite extended sensory deficit, without dermatomal distribution, which is also typical. Such pain has similarities with phantom limb pain: similar to amputees, patients with complete brachial avulsion may experience phantom limb sensation and phantom limb pain and should be questioned about these symptoms.

This man also reports a second less severe pain at the shoulder, which extends to the arm and forearm. This pain is continuous during daytime, described as deep aching. It has no neuropathic characteristics (in particular, no burning, electric shocks, allodynia, tingling, or pins and needles). It is increased by everyday activity and relieved by wearing a sling. This suggests musculoskeletal pain related to muscle impairment. Nonneuropathic pain is very common after BPA and includes mainly musculoskeletal pain related to shoulder subluxation, joint disease, or myofascial

---

BOX 20.1 **Brachial Plexus Avulsion**

BPA is an injury caused by high-energy traction to the brachial plexus, usually during a motorcycle accident, leading to tearing of the spinal nerves from their insertion into the spinal cord.

The site of injury is proximal to the dorsal root ganglia (i.e., preganglionic), but the spinal cord is often injured. BPA may affect the fifth cervical to the first thoracic segments in varying degrees, leading to partial or complete motor, autonomic, and sensory deficits of the upper limb.

A large proportion of BPA patients develop chronic neuropathic pain, which may start from the onset of injury or be delayed by up to several years after the accident and is generally described as paroxysmal (electric shocks).

Treatment should follow international guidelines for neuropathic pain (particularly gabapentin, pregabalin, duloxetine, tricyclic antidepressants, tramadol as second line, and strong opioids as last choice).

In severe refractory cases, the more traditional surgical approach is DREZtomy (lesion of the dorsal root entry zone corresponding to the Lissauer's tract and posterior part of the spinal cord dorsal horn).

---

pain. This pain is frequently perceived at a distant location from the site of injury, here the arm and forearm. Thus, the area of pain may be similar to that of neuropathic pain after BPA, hence the importance of asking patients to describe their pain quality (screening questionnaires are useful here; see Chapter 1).

This patient has several types of pain following BPA, but the worse pain is neuropathic. Neuropathic pain management in this case should follow current international guidelines (Box 20.1), but pain after BPA is generally more difficult to treat than other neuropathic pains (Chapter 2). Here, antiepileptics (gabapentin 1200–2400 mg per day, pregabalin 150–600 mg per day) and antidepressants (tricyclic antidepressants such as amitriptyline, desipramine, or nortriptyline 10–150 mg per day, serotonin–norepinephrine reuptake inhibitor antidepressants such as duloxetine 60–120 mg per day) are recommended. In contrast, topical treatments (lidocaine patches, high-concentration capsaicin plasters) are less relevant for use because the area of pain is totally anesthetic and these drugs act on peripheral mechanisms. Because this patient did not tolerate amitriptyline, you may consider starting with gabapentin 300 mg per day, titrated up by steps of 300 mg every 4–7 days up to efficacy or side effects, the usual analgesic dosages of gabapentin being 1200–1800 mg in three divided dosages. Monitoring should include central side effects such as somnolence and dizziness, but weight gain and peripheral edema are also common. In contrast, no biological monitoring is required. For his musculoskeletal pain, you should add physical therapy and transcutaneous electrical nerve stimulation, provided that the shoulder is not totally anesthetic. If the patient does not tolerate or does not respond to gabapentin, you may switch to pregabalin (this may be done progressively by tapering off the first drug while increasing the second) or duloxetine, or subsequently combine both drugs (e.g., gabapentin or pregabalin with duloxetine).

This patient received gabapentin titrated to 1800 mg in three divided dosages combined with physical therapy by a physiotherapist with modest efficacy (20%) on his pain paroxysms but could not increase the dosages because of somnolence. In contrast, his shoulder pain significantly improved with physical therapy. He then tried pregabalin and duloxetine, but he did not tolerate them and preferred gabapentin. Tramadol and strong opioids, indicated respectively as second and third line in neuropathic pain, were discouraged in this young man, and he was referred to a specialized center. Specialists may also consider the (off-label) use of subcutaneous botulinum toxin A (Chapter 8) and of noninvasive neuromodulatory approaches such as repetitive transcranial magnetic stimulation (rTMS) of the motor cortex (Chapter 41). In severe refractory cases, the more traditional surgical approach is DREZtomy (Chapter 42): this refers to a lesion of the dorsal root entry zone (corresponding to the Lissauer's tract and posterior part of the spinal cord dorsal horn). Based mainly on uncontrolled studies, it seems to provide 75–100% pain reduction in approximately 70% of patients and is more effective in predominant paroxysmal pain. It should only be performed by highly experienced surgeons to decrease the risk of injury of motor tracts within the spinal cord with subsequent motor weakness.

This patient received 10 repeated sessions of rTMS of the motor cortex, with additional excellent efficacy on his pain paroxysms (70%) and continued gabapentin.

KEY POINTS TO REMEMBER

- BPA is caused by high-energy traction to the brachial plexus, usually during a motorcycle accident.
- BPA commonly causes neuropathic (mainly paroxysmal) pain and musculoskeletal pain.
- Neuropathic pain and musculoskeletal pain may be difficult to differentiate in these patients, and this may be aided by screening questionnaires.

Further Reading

Bordalo-Rodrigues M, Siqueira MG, Kurimori CO, et al. Diagnostic accuracy of imaging studies for diagnosing root avulsions in post-traumatic upper brachial plexus traction injuries in adults. *Acta Neurochir.* 2020;162(12):3189–3196.

Clifton WE, Stone JJ, Kumar N, Marek T, Spinner RJ. Delayed myelopathy in patients with traumatic preganglionic brachial plexus avulsion injuries. *World Neurosurg.* 2019;122:e1562–e1569.

Martins RS, Siqueira MG, Heise CO, Foroni L, Neto HS, Teixeira MJ. The nerve to the levator scapulae muscle as donor in brachial plexus surgery: An anatomical study and case series. *J Neurosurg.* 2021:1–8.

Martins RS, Siqueira MG, Heise CO, Foroni L, Teixeira MJ. A prospective study comparing single and double fascicular transfer to restore elbow flexion after brachial plexus injury. *Neurosurgery*. 2013;72(5):709–714.

Santana MV, Bina MT, Paz MG, et al. High prevalence of neuropathic pain in the hand of patients with traumatic brachial plexus injury: A cross-sectional study. *Arq Neuropsiquiatr*. 2016;74(11):895–901.

Teixeira MJ, da Paz MG, Bina MT, et al. Neuropathic pain after brachial plexus avulsion—Central and peripheral mechanisms. *BMC Neurol*. 2015;15:73.

21 Pain and Paraplegia

Nadine Attal and Didier Bouhassira

A 37-year-old patient was severely injured during the
Bataclan terror attack in Paris, France, in November
2015 and suffers from post-traumatic stress disorder.
His pain appeared during rehabilitation. Pain is worse
in the lower limbs, described as burning, cold, and
electric shocks, with tingling, numbness, and pins and
needles. He also reports pain at the inner part of the
forearms and hands; muscle cramps and spasms at
the lower limbs; abdominal cramps during defecation;
and low back and shoulder pain (described as aching
and heavy). At examination, he has total paraplegia,
lower limb spasticity with increased tendon reflexes
and Babinski's sign, and anesthesia of the lower limbs
with a T10 level. Examination also shows hypoesthesia
at the inner surface of the hands and several muscle
trigger points in the lower back and shoulders. He
receives oral baclofen for spasticity and trospium
chloride for neurogenic bladder dysfunction but has
not tolerated pregabalin.

What do you do now?

This patient with T10 paraplegia reports several pain areas. The area of maximal pain is the lower limbs: here, pain is described as burning, cold, and electric shocks, and it is associated with tingling, numbness, and pins and needles, which are typical neuropathic pain characteristics. It extends up to the level of injury (T10) in an area of total sensory deficit. This pain is generally referred to as below-level neuropathic pain and is related to central mechanisms (Table 21.1). His second, more bothersome pain involves the inner part of the forearms and hands and is also suggestive of neuropathic pain but is situated above the level of injury: it is usually called above-level neuropathic pain (see Table 21.1). Mechanisms may involve compression of the ulnar nerves because of the frequent use of the wheelchair. The patient also has both low back and shoulder pain, which are probably musculoskeletal and related to overuse or strain; painful spasms that may be related to his lower limbs spasticity despite baclofen; and intermittent abdominal pain certainly due to his bladder dysfunction and constipation (visceral pain) (see Table 21.1). The mechanisms of these multiple pains after spinal cord injury (SCI) may be difficult to untangle because they may cover the same body areas. Hence, screening questionnaires (see Chapter 1) are helpful to differentiate neuropathic pains from these other pains and are validated in SCI.

This patient did not tolerate FDA- and EMA-approved pregabalin as first line. We advise you to try the antidepressant duloxetine (off-label for SCI pain, FDA and EMA approved for diabetic painful neuropathy). This drug may also improve his post-traumatic stress disorder, and this may be conducted in accordance with his psychiatrist. You may start with 30 mg once daily during meal for 1 week, then increase after 1 week up to 60 mg once daily. For his above-level neuropathic pain (which has peripheral mechanisms), you may also add 5 % lidocaine plasters (two plasters per day on the painful area during 12 consecutive hours; off-label). For his musculoskeletal pains, you should prescribe physical therapy, massages, and, subsequently depending on his response, acupuncture and transcutaneous electrical nerve stimulation (TENS). Last, because he also suffers from painful spasms despite baclofen, we advise you to increase the dosage of baclofen, which is probably underdosed, to three to six tablets per day. If spasticity is refractory, you may send him to a physical therapist, who will consider intramuscular botulinum toxin A if the spasticity is

TABLE 21.1 International Classification of Spinal Cord Injury Pain[a]

Pain Mechanism	Pain Types	Mechanisms
Nociceptive	Musculoskeletal	Bone, joints, trauma, inflammation, mechanical instability, muscle contractions, overuse syndrome
	Visceral	Kidney stone, intestinal disorders, sphincter disorders, etc. Dysautonomic headache
Neuropathic	Above level	Compressive mononeuropathy Complex regional pain syndrome
	At level	Radicular compression (including cauda equina syndrome) Syringomyelia (commonly delayed) Intramedullary tumor Spinal and radicular lesion
	Below level	Spinal trauma/ischemia Phantom sensation

(The left column includes a body silhouette diagram labeled "Above-level pain," "At-level pain," and "Below-level pain.")

[a]Above-level neuropathic pain is peripheral and not directly related to the spinal cord lesion. It is generally due to compression of the ulnar nerves because of the wheelchair. At-level pain may be caused by the spinal cord injury itself (central) or nerve root lesions (peripheral). Below-level pain is purely central, caused by the spinal cord injury, and may be delayed by several years. Mechanisms involve abnormal neuronal excitability rostral to the level of injury and cortical reorganization (as for phantom limb pain). It is often aggravated by triggers such as urinary infection or bedsores. Sensory hypersensitivity (allodynia and hyperalgesia) soon after the injury may predict its late development (supporting a role of neuronal hyperexcitability in this pain).

Adapted from Siddall et al. (2002).

localized, nabiximols (available in several countries), or intrathecal baclofen. Abdominal pain in SCI may be extremely difficult to treat, and the best treatment is that for constipation, which is often the main cause. Here, you may simply add an oral soft laxative such as macrogol to his treatment. Of note, tricyclic antidepressants and opioids, are difficult to use in this patient because he is at high risk of constipation, urinary retention, sweating, and weight gain.

Chronic pain is one of the most disabling consequences of spinal cord injury (SCI), with neuropathic pain affecting approximately 60% of patients. Its management should be multimodal. Nonneuropathic SCI pain encompasses the treatment of spasticity-induced pain with baclofen or botulinum toxin A (for localized spasticity), musculoskeletal pain with analgesics, physical therapy and TENS, and visceral pain with laxatives as the latter is generally related to constipation. For below-level neuropathic pain (central), oral antineuropathic drugs are recommended, akin to other neuropathic pain states (Chapter 2). They include gabapentin 1200–2400 mg per day, pregabalin 150–600 mg per day, tricyclic antidepressants such as amitriptyline 10–150 mg per day, and duloxetine 60–10 mg per day as first line, and tramadol (SR: 100–400 mg per day) as second line. Treatment may also include physical therapies with techniques based on movement illusion and virtual reality (Chapter 30). For at-level (peripheral/central) or above-level SCI (peripheral), additional treatments may include topical agents (5% lidocaine plasters and capsaicin high-concentration patches) (Chapter 28) and transcutaneous electrical nerve stimulation (Chapter 33). Refractory cases of neuropathic SCI pain may necessitate strong opioids (although the latter are often poorly tolerated because of their risk of constipation and dysuria), brain neurostimulation techniques such as rTMS of the motor cortex, and for more severe cases intrathecal therapy with morphine or ziconotide (Chapter 45).

KEY POINTS TO REMEMBER

- Pain after SCI is frequent and often neuropathic, but other types of pain (e.g., musculoskeletal, spasticity, viscreral pain) often coexist.
- Screening questionnaires such as DN4, PainDETECT, or LANSS are helpful to discriminate neuropathic SCI pain from these other types of pain.

- The management of SCI pain should be multimodal and depend on pain mechanisms. For below-level neuropathic pain (central), oral antineuropathic drugs (gabapentinoids, tricyclic antidepressants, duloxetine, and tramadol) and physical therapies including techniques based on movement illusion and virtual reality may be proposed. For at-level (peripheral/central) or above-level SCI (peripheral), additional treatments may include topical agents (lidocaine plasters and capsaicin high-concentration patches) and TENS.

Further Reading

Attal N. Spinal cord injury pain. *Rev Neurol*. 2021;177:606–612.

Austin PD, Siddall PJ. Virtual reality for the treatment of neuropathic pain in people with spinal cord injuries: A scoping review. *J Spinal Cord Med*. 2021;44(1):8–18.

Bryce TN, Biering-Sorensen F, Finnerup NB, et al. International Spinal Cord Injury Pain (ISCIP) classification: Part I. Background and description. *Spinal Cord*. 2012;50:413–417.

Finnerup NB. Pain in patients with spinal cord injury. *Pain*. 2013;154:S71–S76

Finnerup NB, Norrbrink C, Trok K, et al. Phenotypes and predictors of pain following traumatic spinal cord injury: A prospective study. *J Pain*. 2014;15:40–48.

Hunt C, Moman R, Peterson A, et al. Prevalence of chronic pain after spinal cord injury: A systematic review and meta-analysis. *Reg Anesth Pain Med*. 2021;46:328–336.

Quesada C, Pommier B, Fauchon C, et al. New procedure of high-frequency repetitive transcranial magnetic stimulation for central neuropathic pain: A placebo-controlled randomized crossover study. *Pain*. 2020;161:718–728.

Soler MD, Kumru H, Pelayo R, et al. Effectiveness of transcranial direct current stimulation and visual illusion on neuropathic pain in spinal cord injury. *Brain*. 2010;133:2565–2577.

Zeilig G, Enosh S, Rubin-Asher D, Lehr B, Defrin R. The nature and course of sensory changes following spinal cord injury: Predictive properties and implications on the mechanism of central pain. *Brain* 2012;135:418–430.

22 Pain and Multiple Sclerosis

Xavier Moisset

A 48-year-old woman with (MS) reports pain of the lower limbs. Her MS started at age 26 years with an optic neuritis. A few years later, she developed cervical myelitis (confirmed by magnetic resonance imaging). For more than 3 years now, she has suffered from lower limb weakness and fatigue associated with muscle spasms or cramps and stiffness. She reports that these symptoms are increased in case of intense fatigue and even more during urinary tract infections. During the past 2 weeks, she has also presented with sudden, brief (<2 minutes), and extremely painful episodic spasms of the right leg occurring several times a day. These episodes are not associated with loss of consciousness and are triggered by physical activity, considerably impacting daily living activities. She has received duloxetine 60 mg per day for her pain but reports no efficacy.

What do you do now?

This woman has MS with cervical myelitis (Figure 22.1), which started 20 years ago. She is in significant pain. Does she suffer from neuropathic pain? She reports episodic severe sudden and brief painful spasms of the right leg but no other symptoms suggestive of neuropathic pain. Her pain is associated with fatigue, lower limb weakness, and muscle cramps. At examination, there is increased muscle tone and brisk deep tendon reflexes at the lower limbs with Babinski sign, without sensory deficit in the painful area.

Thus, in this woman with MS, pain is not neuropathic. Rather, it corresponds to spasticity-induced pain and painful tonic spasms. Here, the presence of suggestive symptoms (episodic severe sudden and brief painful spasms of the right leg) and signs (increased muscle tone and brisk deep tendon reflexes at the lower limbs with Babinski sign) and lack of neuropathic characteristics of the pain orient toward this diagnosis.

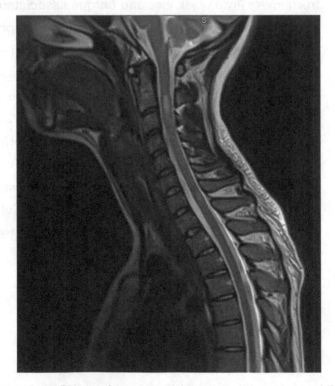

FIGURE 22.1 Sagittal T2 image of the spinal cord showing a cervical myelitis due to MS.

Although frequent, neuropathic pain is not the only pain type observed in patients with MS (Table 22.1). For this woman, you should first discontinue duloxetine, which is ineffective (she may reduce the dosage to 30 mg for 1 week before stopping the drug). For her spasticity (Table 22.2), you may start with U.S. Food and Drug Administration (FDA)/European Medicines Agency (EMA) approved oral baclofen 200 mg per day and then titrate it up to 600–1200 mg per day, depending on efficacy and tolerabilty.

TABLE 22.1 **Pain Types Associated with Multiple Sclerosis**

Neuropathic pain	30% of cases. Continuous (mainly involving extremities) or paroxysmal (unilateral or bilateral trigeminal neuralgia) Lesions: somatosensory lesions in the spinal cord (myelitis), brain (++ brainstem), or both. Associated with more severe MS outcome, but may also occur early
Spasticity	30% of cases. Abnormal increase in muscle tone or stiffness, interfering with movement or associated with discomfort/pain Lesions: upper motor neurons of the corticospinal tract (results in abnormal supraspinal driving of spinal reflexes) Tonic spasticity (stiffness, hypertonicity): increased muscle tone, assessed by the resistance during passive soft tissue stretching (modified Ashworth scale) Phasic spasticity (muscle spasms): reproduced by hyperventilation (wide and quicker respiratory movements for 1 or 2 min) Clonus (rapid muscle contractions)
Painful tonic spasms	Corresponds to paroxysmal dystonia Brief muscle contractions (30 sec to 3 min). Without impaired consciousness (normal electroencephalogram) usually triggered by hyperventilation Lesions: motor pathways (internal capsule, cerebral peduncle, or spinal cord)
Headache	Migraine or tension-type headache. Common in young women but prevalence doubled in multiple sclerosis

TABLE 22.2 **Modified Ashworth Scale**

0	No increase in muscle tone
1	Slight increase in muscle tone, manifested by a catch and release or by minimal resistance at the end of the range of motion when the affected part(s) is moved in flexion or extension
1+	Slight increase in muscle tone, manifested by a catch, followed by minimal resistance throughout the remainder (less than half) of the range of motion
2	More marked increase in muscle tone through most of the range of motion, but affected part(s) easily moved
3	Considerable increase in muscle tone; passive movement difficult
4	Affected part(s) rigid in flexion or extension

Other therapeutic options include FDA/EMA approved oral tizanidine, an α_2-adrenergic receptor agonist (usual dose 8–36 mg a day TID, starting with 4 mg at night) or oral gabapentin (off-label for spasticity), which may also be titrated from 300 mg per day to 800–900 mg per day (maximal dosage 3600 mg per day). Regarding her painful spasms, you may try carbamazepine (200 per day in the evening and then titrate up by steps of 200 mg every 4 days to 600–1200 mg per day) or oxcarbazepine 300–2400 mg because response to these drugs is generally excellent (although no high-quality randomized controlled trials have confirmed their efficacy). If spasticity does not respond to these options, you may refer this patient to a specialized center for treatments such as diazepam, dantrolene, oromucosal nabiximols (provided that they are available), or intramuscular injections of botulinum toxin A (particularly if spasticity is localized) and then intrathecal baclofen. Repetitive transcranial magnetic stimulation of the motor cortex may also induce some benefit. For refractory painful tonic spasms, other antiepileptics (lamotrigine or gabapentinoids), acetazolamide, and botulinum toxin A may also be useful.

This woman was treated by oral baclofen titrated up to 600 mg per day, but dosages could not be increased further because of somnolence. Oral tizanidine was initiated at 4 mg per day and titrated to 16 mg per day. This combination substantially relieved her spasticity-induced pain (by 70%) but not her tonic spasms, which were further treated by a neurologist with carbamazepine 800 mg per day.

- Patients with MS report multiple pain types, including neuropathic pain and migraine, but also spasticity and painful tonic spasms.
- Spasticity can be evaluated using the modified Ashworth scale.
- Painful tonic spasms can be induced/reproduced by hyperventilation.
- The treatment of spasticity relies on oral baclofen, tizanidine, gabapentin, and, for more refractory cases, oromucosal spray of nabiximols.
- Painful tonic spasms are well controlled using sodium channel blockers such as carbamazepine and oxcarbazepine.

Further Reading

Comi G, Solari A, Leocani L, Centonze D, Otero-Romero S; Italian Consensus Group on Treatment of Spasticity in Multiple Sclerosis. Italian consensus on treatment of spasticity in multiple sclerosis. *Eur J Neurol.* 2020;27(3):445–453.

June 17, 2013 e-pearl of the week: Tonic spasms. *Neurology.* 2013. https://n.neurology. org/epearls/20130617. Accessed July 16, 2021.

Moisset X, Giraud P, Dallel R. Migraine in multiple sclerosis and other chronic inflammatory diseases. *Rev Neurol (Paris).* 2021 Sep;177(7):816–820.

Otero-Romero S, Sastre-Garriga J, Comi G, et al. Pharmacological management of spasticity in multiple sclerosis: Systematic review and consensus paper. *Mult Scler.* 2016;22(11):1386–1396.

Solaro C, Cella M, Signori A, et al.; Neuropathic Pain Special Interest Group of the Italian Neurological Society. Identifying neuropathic pain in patients with multiple sclerosis: A cross-sectional multicenter study using highly specific criteria. *J Neurol.* 2018;265(4):828–835.

Spissu A, Cannas A, Ferrigno P, Pelaghi AE, Spissu M. Anatomic correlates of painful tonic spasms in multiple sclerosis. *Mov Disord.* 1999;14(2):331–335.

23 Sudden-Onset Facial Pain

Sandra Sif Gylfadottir and
Nanna Brix Finnerup

A 78-year-old man with a past medical history of
hypertension, hyperlipidemia, and type 2 diabetes
presents with left-sided periorbital facial pain. Three
months ago, he suddenly experienced unsteady
gait, nausea, and numbness in the left side of the
face. Within a month, he developed left facial pain,
concentrated around the eye, described as continuous,
burning, and stabbing and associated with tingling.
There are no relieving or aggravating factors.
He also complains of unpleasant sensation and
hypersensitivity to light touch in the right arm and leg.
Neurological examination reveals reduced sensation
for pinprick and temperature in the whole left hemiface
and reduced pinprick sensation and evoked pain
to brush (allodynia) in the right arm and leg. There
is no vibration or touch deficit, no impairment of
proprioception, and motor tone is normal, as are
tendon reflexes. Gabapentin 300 mg BID was initiated
and induced minor improvement of pain intensity.

What do you do now?

This patient complains of periorbital pain. To orient the diagnosis, you need to obtain a detailed pain history and description and assess the relieving or aggravating factors (e.g., eating, cold/hot weather, and light touch) and the presence of associated symptoms, such as other pains and other symptoms in the face (redness of the eye, tearing, and altered sensation).

The patient describes his facial pain as continuous (burning and stabbing), associated with tingling, which suggests neuropathic quality. This may be confirmed by screening questionnaires (see Chapter 1). Pain has a periorbital distribution and a sudden onset, but it is not described as paroxysmal (no electric shocks), its intensity is moderate, there are no triggers for the pain (e.g., brushing teeth, eating, or swallowing), and there is no redness of the face. This seems to rule out trigeminal neuralgia and cluster headache (Table 23.1, see also Chapter 18). Importantly the patient also complains of unsteady gait, which suggests a central lesion.

Clinical examination is mandatory. It reveals reduced sensation for pinprick and temperature on the whole left hemiface, and reduced pinprick sensation and evoked pain to brush (allodynia) in the opposite arm and leg. This presentation (facial trigeminal pain and hypoesthesia, and contralateral hypoesthesia to pinprick in the limbs) is typical of crossed brainstem syndrome. Facial pain may be associated with ipsilateral Horner syndrome; cerebellar and vestibular syndrome; and ipsilateral impairment of the 9th, 10th, and 11th cranial nerves (sensory deficit of the posterior one-third of the tongue, dysphagia, swallowing difficulties, nasal speech, and regurgitation of liquids through the nose).

Based on the sudden onset of symptoms, pain in the same area soon thereafter, age, and comorbidity with more than one vascular risk factors, the most probable diagnosis is central post-stroke pain (CPSP). To confirm the diagnosis, you need to ask for magnetic resonance imaging (MRI) of the brain. MRI showed a recent left-sided dorsal lateral medullary infarction (Figure 23.1). Thus, the diagnosis is neuropathic post-stroke (facial) pain due to dorsolateral medullary infarction, also called Wallenberg syndrome.

You should first initiate antiplatelet therapy together with assessment of risk factors for stroke. You may ask for evaluation and management

TABLE 23.1 Main Causes of Unilateral Facial Pain and Their Clinical Characteristics

Cluster headache	Attacks of severe, strictly unilateral pain which is orbital, supraorbital, temporal or in any combination of these sites, lasting 15–180 minutes and occurring from once every other day to eight times a day. Associated with ipsilateral conjunctival injection, lacrimation, nasal congestion, rhinorrhoea, forehead and facial sweating, miosis, ptosis and/or eyelid oedema, and/or with restlessness or agitation
Trigeminal neuralgia (classical, idiopathic)	Recurrent unilateral brief electric shock-like pains, abrupt in onset and termination (paroxysmal), limited to the distribution of one or more divisions of the trigeminal nerve and triggered by innocuous stimuli (brushing the teeth, eating, speaking)
Migraine	Attacks lasting 4–72 hours. Unilateral location, pulsating quality, moderate or severe intensity, aggravation by routine physical activity Association with nausea and/or photophobia and phonophobia
Rhinosinusitis	In temporal relation to the onset and outcome of rhinosinusitis Exacerbated by pressure over the paranasal sinusesi
Giant cell arteritis (GCA)	Temporal relation to onset and outcome of GCA, or has led to the diagnosis of GCA Associated with scalp tenderness and/or jaw claudication
Optic neuritis	Unilateral or bilateral retro-orbital, orbital, frontal and/or temporal pain Temporal relation to the optic neuritis Pain aggravated by eye movement
Disorder of the teeth	Temporal relation to the onset and outcome of the disorder or appearance of the lesion Exacerbated by palpation, probing or pressure applied to the affected tooth or teeth

(*continued*)

TABLE 23.1 **Continued**

Headache attributed to temporomandibular disorder (TMD)	Temporal relation to temporomandibular disorder Aggravated by jaw motion, jaw function (e.g., chewing) and/or jaw parafunction (e.g., bruxism) Provoked on physical examination by temporalis muscle palpation and/or passive movement of the jaw
Post herpetic neuralgia	Unilateral facial pain in the distribution(s) of a trigeminal nerve branch or branches, persisting or recurring for >3 months with temporal relation to the herpes zoster infection

by a physical therapist because of gait instability. Regarding neuropathic pain, you have the choice as first line of pregabalin, gabapentin, tricyclic antidepressants (amitriptyline and nortriptyline), and serotonin–noradrenaline reuptake inhibitors (e.g., duloxetine); topical agents have no place in post-stroke pain. None has specific approval for use in

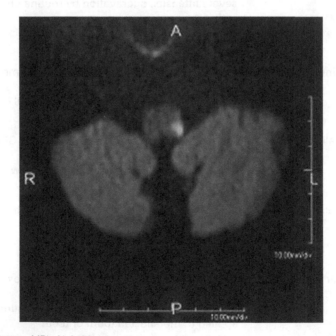

FIGURE 23.1 MRI of left-sided dorsal lateral medullary stroke.

post-stroke pain, but they are approved for other neuropathic pains, and pregabalin in particular is U.S. Food and Drug Administration approved for another type of central pain (spinal cord injury pain) (see Chapter 2). Of note, the efficacy of opioids is generally weak in post-stroke pain. Regarding other pain syndromes, musculoskeletal pain may necessitate physical therapy, whereas painful spasticity may be treated by oral baclofen or botulinum toxin A intramuscular injections (if it is localized) in specialist settings.

This patient receives gabapentin, but dosages are small. With lack of renal failure, the best strategy is to increase gabapentin by steps of 300 mg each week to 600 mg three times daily. This patient increased gabapentin up to 1800 mg with additional effect on pain (30%), but doses could not be increased further because of dizziness and drowsiness. Six months later, he visits you again because his pain is becoming intolerable and he has difficulty falling asleep. You may then add nortriptyline 10 mg tablets after checking electrocardiogram to evaluate the QT interval—that is, nortriptyline one tablet for 1 week and then increase gradually by steps of one tablet per week for up to 50 mg or less depending on efficacy or side effects (doses will be difficult to increase further because of potential cardiac toxicity and age, although nortriptyline has less cardiotoxicity than amitriptyline and imipramine). You should reach the recommended dose of each drug before trying another and, if necessary, combine drugs with different modes of action (gabapentin and pregabalin should not be combined). Because this patient has difficulty coping with pain, you should ask for psychological management.

CPSP is a neuropathic pain occurring after hemorrhagic or ischemic stroke (10% of cases; in up to 25% of cases, the pain occurs after thalamic or medullary stroke) caused by a central lesion of the somatosensory pathways. It can arise at the acute stage or be delayed by weeks to months. Characteristic features are similar to those of other neuropathic pains. Diagnosis should be based on history of stroke, pain occurring with a temporal relationship with the stroke, and sensory deficit in the body area corresponding to the brain lesion. Confirmatory tests necessitate neuroimaging. Exclusion of other causes of pain (musculoskeletal, headache, or spasticity) may be helped by screening questionnaires.

- Facial pain associated with other neurological symptoms and findings should warrant an MRI of the central nervous system.
- Ipsilateral facial pain is often seen in Wallenberg syndrome, one of the well-established causes of CPSP (generally caused by occlusion of the vertebral artery at the dorsolateral medulla). Clinicians should be aware of this typical complication.
- The symptoms of central post-stroke pain are similar to those of other types of neuropathic pain, and the treatment is based on evidence-based recommendations for the treatment of neuropathic pain.

Further Reading

Finnerup NB, Attal N, Haroutounian S, et al. Pharmacotherapy for neuropathic pain in adults: A systematic review and meta-analysis. *Lancet Neurol.* 2015;14(2):162–173.

Finnerup NB, Haroutounian S, Kamerman P, et al. Neuropathic pain: An updated grading system for research and clinical practice. *Pain.* 2016;157(8):1599–1606.

Fitzek S, Baumgärtner U, Fitzek C, et al. Mechanisms and predictors of chronic facial pain in lateral medullary infarction. *Ann Neurol.* 2001;49(4):493–500.

Klit H, Finnerup NB, Jensen TS. Central post-stroke pain: Clinical characteristics, pathophysiology, and management. *Lancet Neurol.* 2009;8(9):857–868.

Liampas A, Velidakis N, Georgiou T, et al. Prevalence and management challenges in central post-stroke neuropathic pain: A systematic review and meta-analysis. *Adv Ther.* 2020;37(7):3278–3291.

Mizumoto J. Central poststroke pain with Wallenberg syndrome. *Am J Med.* 2020;133(1):e11–e12.

Ravichandran A, Elsayed KS, Yacoub HA. Central pain mimicking trigeminal neuralgia as a result of lateral medullary ischemic stroke. *Case Rep Neurol Med* 2019;2019:4235724.

Zakrzewska JM. Differential diagnosis of facial pain and guidelines for management. *Br J Anaesth.* 2013;111(1):95–104.

24 Pain and Parkinson Disease

Xavier Moisset

An 82-year-old man with Parkinson disease (PD) for 10 years reports various pain types. He mainly complains of right painful shoulder (his worst pain) associated with stiffness and loss of range of movement that started 12 years ago. This shoulder pain was present at least 2 years before his physician diagnosed PD. It is described as squeezing and cramping, and it is associated with stiffness and loss of range of movement. Pain was initially improved when he started levodopa, but it reappeared 2 years ago. Now it is present especially in the morning before he takes levodopa. The patient also reports episodes of painful curling of the toes particularly while walking, which predominates on the right side. It is most commonly increased during off periods and at walking. Finally, he complains of axial low back and neck pain, which is more moderate, present almost continuously. At examination, there is parkinsonian syndrome with rigidity and akinesia, which predominates on the right side of the body.

What do you do now?

Pain is frequent in PD (approximately two-thirds of patients) and is one of the most common and troublesome nonmotor symptoms. It can appear at any time during the disease and may be present before diagnosis. This patient with PD suffers from several types of pain (Figure 24.1). The first question to ask him is whether there is any relationship (chronological or topographical) between his PD and pain. Because he reports several pain problems, it is advised to start with his most bothersome pain, which is his shoulder pain. His shoulder pain was present at least 2 years before the diagnosis of PD. Pain was initially improved when he started levodopa, but it reappeared 2 years ago. Now it is present especially in the morning before he takes levodopa. It is located on the right shoulder, where his stiffness is worse. This suggests that his shoulder pain is PD related. The second question is how he describes his shoulder pain and whether there are associated

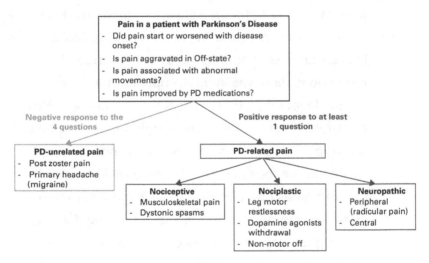

FIGURE 24.1 Classification of pain in patients with PD.

Nociceptive PD-related pain is the most frequent pain type and includes musculoskeletal pain and dystonic pain. Nociplastic PD-related pain is defined as pain that arises from altered nociception despite no clear evidence for actual or threatened tissue damage or for disease or lesion of the somatosensory system. Leg motor restlessness in PD is the most frequent. Neuropathic PD-related pain can be peripheral (e.g., radicular pain) or central. PD-unrelated pain corresponds to pain that is neither caused nor aggravated by the disease, such as osteoarthritis, primary headache, or postherpetic neuralgia.

Adapted from Mylius et al. (2021).

symptoms. His shoulder pain is described as squeezing and cramping and is associated with stiffness and loss of range of movement. Thus, it has no neuropathic characteristics. Shoulder pain is one of the symptoms that can lead to the diagnosis of PD and often precedes the diagnosis. It is sometimes misdiagnosed as a frozen shoulder. It can be improved by dopaminergic treatments and can recur or increase in "off" periods, as is the case for tremor and rigidity.

This man reports a second type of pain, which involves the toe, with painful intermittent episodes of curling and clenched toes. As is the case for shoulder pain, this toe pain predominates on the right side, where motor symptoms predominate. It is most commonly increased during off periods and at walking. There are no other symptoms. This second pain type also probably corresponds to PD-related pain. Here, the description of the pain is characteristic of dystonia, which also corresponds to nociceptive pain. Dystonia refers to uncontrolled and often painful muscle movements (spasms). They are often twisting or turning movements, such as toe dorsiflexion or foot inversion and/or plantar flexion. These involuntary movements can impair gait and cause cramping and aching pain. Dystonia is sometimes precipitated or worsened by voluntary actions, such as walking. It generally occurs later than other pain symptoms during the evolution of PD. It can be increased by off-time because muscular stiffness increases mechanical strains. Abnormal stresses on joints, especially on the spine, can lead to mechanical pain or an increase in a pre-existing pain, for example, due to osteoarthritis. The manifestations of dystonia in PD also include blepharospasm, torticolis, upper extremity flexion and adduction, camptocormia, and Pisa syndrome (also called pleurothotonus; reversible lateral bending of the trunk with a tendency to lean to one side).

Finally, this man also reports chronic low back and neck pain. This third type of pain does not seem to be related to his PD because it is not worse in off periods, it is axial, and it does not predominate on the side where motor symptoms are worse. It should be kept in mind that low back pain, which is also nociceptive pain, is the most frequent chronic pain problem in the general population, particularly at this patient's age. Such pain is even more frequent and severe in PD patients, probably due to the stooped posture that increases mechanical strains. Other PD-unrelated pain (pain that is neither caused nor aggravated by the disease) includes osteoarthritis, low back pain, primary headache, or postherpetic neuralgia.

This clinical case illustrates the three most common pain conditions observed in patients with PD, here all of nociceptive types. However, PD patients may also suffer from neuropathic and nociplastic pains that can be related or unrelated to their PD. Neuropathic PD-related pain can be peripheral (e.g., radicular pain) or central. The latter, also called Parkinsonian central pain (PCP) or primary pain is generally poorly defined and may not resemble other types of central pains (such as post-stroke or spinal cord injury pains). It is often diffuse, bilateral, or predominates on the side where motor symptoms occurred. It may have a dysautonomic character, with visceral sensations or dyspnea, and may vary in parallel with the levodopa medications as a nonmotor fluctuation. It is not explained by rigidity, dystonia, and musculoskeletal or internal organ lesions. Screening questionnaires validated for neuropathic pain are not relevant here, and there is no validated scale for the diagnosis, which often remains one of exclusion. Nociplastic PD-related pain ("pain that arises from altered nociception despite no clear evidence for actual or threatened tissue damage or for disease or lesion of the somatosensory system") includes in particular restless leg syndrome (Box 24.1).

How do you manage this patient? You will probably find it easier to manage his unrelated PD low back and neck pain. You may use conventional step 1 analgesics, possibly nonsteroidal anti-inflammatory drugs for short periods of time, physical therapy, massages, and transcutaneous electrical nerve stimulation. Regarding his PD-related dystonia and spasms, you should refer this patient to a specialist in order to optimize the dopaminergic treatment. For all PD-related pains, optimizing the dopaminergic treatment can indeed help reduce mechanical strains when reducing off periods. It can be useful to increase the overall daily dose of levodopa or dopamine agonists, dividing the doses while increasing the frequency of dosing. For refractory cases, deep brain stimulation (DBS) targeting the subthalamic nucleus has been shown to improve pain, independently from motor improvement. After DBS, pain alleviation might be attributable to a direct central modulation of pain perception.

The management of Parkinsonien central pain is difficult. If this pain does not respond to dopaminergic adaptation, antineuropathis agents, including antidepressants such as tricyclic antidepressants (preferably at low dosages), duloxetine, and gabapentin or pregabalin may be used, but they may be poorly tolerated in patients with PD.

KEY POINTS TO REMEMBER

- Pain is a common nonmotor symptom in patients with PD.
- Pain can appear at any time during the disease and is often present before diagnosis.
- Pain can be PD-related or PD-unrelated and is more commonly nociceptive than neuropathic
- PD-related pain is generally worsened in off-state and can be improved by optimization of dopamine treatment.

Further Reading

Marques A, Attal N, Bouhassira D, et al. How to diagnose parkinsonian central pain? *Parkinsonism Relat Disord*. 2019;64:50–53.

Mylius V, Perez Lloret S, Cury RG, et al. The Parkinson disease pain classification system: Results from an international mechanism-based classification approach. *Pain*. 2021;162(4):1201–1210.

25 Red Feet and Hands

David LH Bennett and
Andreas Themistocleous

A 20-year-old woman comes in consultation because
of red feet. She tells you that her mother had noted
that she had red feet from the age of 1 year, and
as long as she can remember, she had episodes of
burning pain in the feet. These were associated with
erythema and triggered by warmth, and cooling the
feet (e.g., in water) could help relieve the episodes.
The episodes became more frequent when she was
a teenager. Because she was often putting her feet
in freezing water, she developed skin ulceration
necessitating hospital admission. As she became
older, she also developed erythema and pain of her
fingers and ears. Her father had suffered from similar
symptoms. Clinical examination shows strictly no
sensory impairment, tendon reflexes are normal, and
there is no motor deficit, but there is clear evidence
for erythema of the feet. Her pain is poorly relieved by
codeine combined with acetaminophen.

What do you do now?

This 20-year-old woman complains of erythema of the feet and then fingers and ears triggered by warm and improved by cold, which started when she was age 1 year. She also reports neuropathic type of pain (burning feet). A sensory neuropathy might be discussed, but sensory examination was normal, and this pain evoked exclusively by heat and associated with red feet is uncommon in sensory neuropathies. For this young woman, the most likely diagnosis is erythromelalgia. Erythromelalgia (*erythrose*, redness; *melos*, extremity; *algos*, pain; first description by S. Weir Mitchell in 1878) is a rare condition characterized by episodic burning pain and erythema of the distal extremities (i.e., feet and hands), less commonly proximal the hands, arms, legs, ears, and face. Warmth, exercise, enclosed shoes, alcohol, and spicy foods often precipitate pain attacks that can be partially relieved by cooling. The diagnosis is clinical, based on the nature of symptoms, young age, and normal clinical examination (Figure 25.1).

Erythromelalgia may be primary or secondary to multiple causes (e.g., myeloproliferative diseases, autoimmune disorders, small fiber neuropathy, vasodilated drugs such as calcium channel blockers, and collagen disorders/joint hypermobility [the most common cause in those younger than age 40 years]). You should first conduct a sensory examination searching for deficits to pinprick and temperature to rule out neuropathy. In case of deficits, complementary investigations (see Chapter 38) are warranted (nerve conduction studies/electromyography, quantitative sensory testing, or skin punch biopsy). Here, sensory examination was strictly normal; therefore, these tests are not necessary. Second, you should ask for screening blood tests, including full blood count, an autoimmune screen, coagulation screen, hemoglobin A1C, plasma protein electrophoresis, C-reactive protein, and erythrocyte sedimentation rate. In this woman, blood tests were normal.

Giving her young age, normal examination and tests, and probable family history (her father had the same symptoms), the most plausible diagnosis is primary (inherited) erythromelalgia. Age of onset is usually within the first two decades, with an autosomal dominant inheritance. However, some patients have de novo mutations, so a negative family history does not exclude the diagnosis. Inherited erythromelalgia is caused by gain-of-function mutations (>20 described thus far) in the gene (*SCN9a*) encoding one specific voltage-gated sodium channel (Nav1.7).

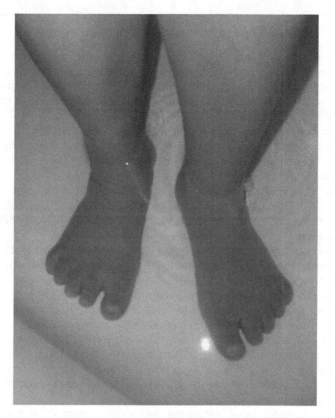

FIGURE 25.1 The erythema of the feet and lower leg of a patient with inherited erythromelalgia. She is standing in cold water in an attempt to reduce her symptoms during a flare.

Neurological examination is normal, but erythema of the feet is usually apparent.

It is mandatory to ask for genetic testing (the format depends on the local health care pathways) in specialized settings because a monogenic pain disorder is suspected (Box 25.1). However, you do not need to wait for results to treat this young woman's symptoms. You should advise her about the dangers of extreme cooling (ice baths), which caused skin ulcers, and suggest alternative strategies such as fans and avoid warming of her feet. Regarding drug therapy, it is still common for these patients to be prescribed opioids, but the latter are inappropriate. Thus, you should progressively taper codeine off, which was not effective. Drug treatments may

- Genetic testing is routinely employed in a minority of cases of neuropathic pain when a monogenic pain disorder is suspected. In this case the clinical phenotype can usually be defined on the clinical history and examination and is characteristic enough to refer for genetic testing.
- The commonest gene that is being investigated is SCN9a (encoding Nav1.7) particularly in relation to painful neuropathies (such as small fibre neuropathy). SCN10a and SCN11a (encoding Nav1.8 and 1.9 respectively) may also be relevant.
- Many genetic centres, including in particular the UK National Health Service, tend to use next generation sequencing techniques and simultaneously sequencing panels of genes. Whole Genome Sequencing is also increasingly undertaken.
- It can be a challenge to determine whether gene variants that have been found are pathogenic. This requires careful thought and genetic counselling.
- Genetic testing can impact on treatment choice. Certain inherited erythromelalgia mutations respond to drugs which block sodium channels such as mexiletine and paroxysmal extreme pain disorder generally responds well to treatment with carbamazepine. The drug lacosamide (which is a blocker of sodium channels) which does not show efficacy in unselected patients did show significant efficacy in patients with small fiber neuropathy and rare variants in Nav1.7.
- Genetic testing is not yet advised in common neuropathic pain disorders (such as painful diabetic neuropathy). As genetic expands it may be possible to use techniques such as polygenic risk score to identify those most at risk of neuropathic pain. This is currently in the research domain but this is a rapidly moving field.

include those recommended for neuropathic pain (pregabalin, gabapentin, duloxetine, and amitriptyline), but they induce many side effects and this woman is very young. Hence, we advise you to treat her with 5% lidocaine plasters (one plaster to cover each foot during 12 hours, off-label) because it is a safe topical agent (no systemic side effects) and blocks sodium channels (involved in erythromelalgia).

Topical lidocaine plasters 5% had 30% efficacy on her symptoms. After a few weeks, results of genetic testing revealed mutations in the *SCN9a* gene. She was referred to a neurologist who treated her with off-label oral mexiletine (a sodium channel blocker), the drug of choice for this condition (but not for other neuropathic pains). Being an antiarrhythmic, mexiletine interferes with cardiac conduction, so pretreatment electrocardiography (ECG) repeated after dose escalation is warranted. In this woman, after checking that ECG was normal, mexiletine was titrated from 200 mg daily to 800 mg per day (BID). She initially complained of dizziness, lightheadedness, and nausea (frequent side effects), but she had no cardiac effects (control ECG was normal), and these effects gradually subsided. She now reports 80% efficacy and acceptable safety of mexiletine combined with topical lidocaine, warm eviction (whenever possible), and frequent use of fans.

Other inherited neuropathic pains include paroxysmal extreme pain disorder, characterized by reddening and pain of a specific body region (the perineum), associated with mandibular and ocular pain. Triggers include mechanical stimulation, and the drug of choice is carbamazepine.

KEY POINTS TO REMEMBER

- Erythromelalgia is a rare condition characterized by episodic burning pain and erythema of the distal extremities.
- Warmth, exercise, enclosed shoes, alcohol, and spicy foods often precipitate pain attacks that can be partially relieved by cooling.
- The diagnosis is clinical, based on the nature of symptoms, young age, erythema and lack of sensory deficit.
- Primary erythromelalgia is genetic, whereas secondary causes include myeloproliferative diseases, autoimmune disorders, small fiber neuropathy, vasodilated drugs, and collagen disorders/joint hypermobility.

Further Reading

Alsaloum, M., Higerd GP, Effraim PR, Waxman SG. Status of peripheral sodium channel blockers for non-addictive pain treatment. *Nat Rev Neurol.* 2020;16(12):689–705.

Bennett DL, Clark AJ, Huang J, Waxman SG, Dib Hajj SD. The role of voltage-gated sodium channels in pain signaling. *Physiol Rev.* 2019;99(2):1079–1151.

Bennett DL, Woods CG. Painful and painless channelopathies. *Lancet Neurol.* 2014;13(6):587–599.

Cook-Norris RH, Tollefson MM, Cruz-Inigo AE, Sandroni P, Davis MDP, Davis MR. Pediatric erythromelalgia: A retrospective review of 32 cases evaluated at Mayo Clinic over a 37-year period. *J Am Acad Dermatol.* 2012;66(3):416–423.

Dib-Hajj SD, Rush AM, Cummins TR, et al. Gain-of-function mutation in Nav1.7 in familial erythromelalgia induces bursting of sensory neurons. *Brain.* 2005;128(Pt 8):1847–1854.

Labau JIR, Estacion M, Tanaka BS, et al. Differential effect of lacosamide on Nav1.7 variants from responsive and non-responsive patients with small fibre neuropathy. *Brain.* 2020;143(3):771–782.

Turro E, Astle WJ, Megy K, et al. Whole-genome sequencing of patients with rare diseases in a national health system. *Nature.* 2020;583(7814):96–102.

Yang Y, Dib-Hajj SD, Zhang J, et al. Structural modelling and mutant cycle analysis predict pharmacoresponsiveness of a Na(V)1.7 mutant channel. *Nat Commun.* 2012;3:1186.

26 Neuropathic Pain in a Child

Nadine Attal and Didier Bouhassira

An 11-year-old girl (height, 140 cm; weight, 34 kg) has
left hip osteosarcoma invading the left lumbar plexus.
She suffers from extreme pain (9/10 on a numeric
rating scale) in the left foot responsible for fatigue,
sleep problems, and anxiety. At interview by her
pediatrician who is qualified in pain, pain is described
as deep aching, squeezing, lancinating, throbbing,
stabbing, and electric shocks. Examination discloses
tactile allodynia in the painful area, hypoalgesia to
pinprick, and hypoesthesia to cold and heat. Her pain
is not relieved by acetaminophen, ibuprofen, and
oxycodone.

What do you do now?

This child with osteosarcoma suffers from severe stabbing, electric shock-like pain, and presents with allodynia in the painful area. Her clinical examination also shows tactile and thermoalgesic deficit. Her pain is probably neuropathic.

As is the case for adults, diagnosis of neuropathic pain in children should be based on sensory descriptors, history, area of pain, and examination (see Chapter 1), but this is highly influenced by age and developmental stage. Screening questionnaires such as DN4, LANSS, or PainDETECT are possible to use in school-aged children or adolescents, but are not formally validated for use in these populations.

You may treat this girl with gabapentin. Although gabapentin is off-label for pain in children, it is recommended for neuropathic pain in this case: The recommended maintenance dose is 40 mg/kg/day in children aged 3 or 4 years and 25–35 mg/kg/day in children aged 5–11 years. Here, you may titrate the drug up to 1200 mg daily. This girl received gabapentin 900 mg per day, which induced moderate efficacy (30%), and then she finally gained 70% benefit with a combination with small dosages of amitriptyline 20 mg daily, which may also be proposed for her neuropathic pain at her age (off-label). Psychotherapy was also proposed. She subsequently was treated by chemotherapy and surgery for her bone cancer with final good recovery and has been in remission since then.

Cancer in children is rare, but it is the main cause of death by disease among children in developed countries. In 2021 in the United States, it was estimated that 15,590 children and adolescents aged 0–19 years would be diagnosed with cancer and 1,780 would die of the disease. Bone osteosarcoma is the leading type of cancer in children and may be responsible for neuropathic pain generally due to plexus lesion, and it may be responsible for nociceptive pain due to bone lesion.

Other causes of neuropathic pain in children include mainly complex regional pain syndrome (CRPS) and genetic diseases (Table 26.1). This pain has a major impact on quality of life and high risk of disability, anxiety, and depression in children. Such emotional impact is also strongly influenced by parental cognitions, behavior, and emotional factors. There are very few therapeutic studies of neuropathic pain in children, and evidence is mostly derived from adult data. The most commonly prescribed treatments

TABLE 26.1 **Common and Uncommon Causes of Chronic Neuropathic Pain in Children[a]**

ICD-11 Classification	Mechanisms of Pain	Description
More common neuropathic pains		
Peripheral nerve injury	Surgery/trauma Cancer-related compression/ infiltration	Phantom pain less common if amputation <6 years Solid tumor (osteosarcoma main condition in children), neurofibromatosis
Painful polyneuropathy	Neurotoxic drugs Autoimmune Genetic/channelopathy Genetic/metabolic	Chemotherapy induced Guillain–Barré syndrome Erythromelalgia Fabry disease
Spinal cord injury	Trauma/tumor	Pain less common than in adults
Brain injury	Tumor	Supra- and infratentorial tumors
Rare or very rare neuropathic pains		
Postherpetic neuralgia	Infection	Very rare in children except immunocompromised
Trigeminal neuralgia	Idiopathic/compression	<2% before age 18 years
Radiculopathy	Nerve root trauma/ tumor	Surgery (e.g., scoliosis) Neuroblastoma
Stroke	Cerebrovascular lesion (infarction, hemorrhage)	Very rare pain in children
Multiple sclerosis		Onset before age 16 years in 2–5% of cases

[a]The table lists the "more common" and "rare or very rare" prevalence of pain caused by the condition but not the condition itself (always rare in children).
Modified from Walker (2020).

(off-label in children) include tricyclic antidepressants (amitriptyline or clomipramine) and gabapentin. Transcutaneous electrical nerve stimulation, capsaicin cream, and eutectic mixture of lidocaine and prilocaine cream have been suggested to be beneficial in anecdotal reports. Physical therapy is recommended for CRPS or neuropathic pain after nerve trauma. Invasive treatments (intrathecal therapy and neurolytic procedures) have been used for severe refractory cases.

KEY POINTS TO REMEMBER

- Main causes of neuropathic pain in children and adolescents include CRPS, cancer, Guillain–Barré syndrome, spinal cord injury, nerve trauma, and genetic conditions.
- Screening questionnaires for neuropathic pain have not been formally validated but may be relevant for use in school-aged children and adolescents.
- Therapy is difficult and mostly extrapolated from adult recommendations, with gabapentin being the drug of choice.

Further Reading

Moisset X, Bouhassira D, Avez Couturier J, et al. Pharmacological and non-pharmacological treatments for neuropathic pain: Systematic review and French recommendations. *Rev Neurol.* 2020;176(5):325–352.

Siegel RL, Miller KD, Fuchs HE, Jemal A. Cancer statistics, 2021. *CA Cancer J Clin.* 2021;71(1):7–33.

Verriotis M, Peters J, Sorger C, Walker SM. Phenotyping peripheral neuropathic pain in male and female adolescents: Pain descriptors, somatosensory profiles, conditioned pain modulation, and child–parent reported disability. *Pain.* 2021;162(6):1732–1748.

Walco GA, Dworkin RH, Krane EJ, et al. Neuropathic pain in children: Special considerations. *Mayo Clin Proc.* 2010;85(3 Suppl):S33–S41.

Walker SM. Neuropathic pain in children: Steps towards improved recognition and management. *EBioMedicine.* 2020;62:103124.

World Health Organization. ICD-11: International classification of diseases. 11th rev. 2019. https://icd.who.int

Common Therapeutic Options

27 Antidepressants and Antiepileptics

Nadine Attal and Didier Bouhassira

A 28-year-old man was in a severe motorbike accident
6 months ago, which resulted in spinal cord injury
with paraparesia. During rehabilitation, he has
started suffering from moderate neuropathic pain of
the lower limbs described mainly as electric shocks
and burning associated with a pricking sensation.
Sensory examination shows near-complete tactile
and thermoalgesic deficit with T10 level. There
is no allodynia. He took acetaminophen during
rehabilitation without any effect and has returned
home. No other drug treatment was proposed. He
states that since he returned home, lower limb pain
has worsened. Pain is now rated as 8/10 on a numeric
rating scale, with pain paroxysms rated as 10/10.
Because pain is responsible for anxiety and sleep
disorders, his physician prescribed fluoxetine 20 mg
daily. This drug has not improved the pain, but the
patient states that he now feels less anxious, although
his sleep is still poor.

What do you do now?

In this young man with spinal cord injury and lower limb pain, antidepressants or antiepileptics such as gabapentin or pregabalin are the drugs of choice because the mechanisms of his pain are central (and these drugs act mainly on central mechanisms). Furthermore, they have anxiolytic effects and may improve sleep. The easiest option is to continue fluoxetine (which improves his anxiety and is well tolerated) and add gabapentin or pregabalin. At his age, it is not mandatory to check for renal insufficiency, but monitoring of potential abuse or misuse is necessary: Gabapentin and pregabalin have mild potential for abuse, and young men are at higher risk of addiction compared to elderly patients. It is advisable to check that this patient does not take higher dosages than prescribed. You may start with U.S. Food and Drug Administration-approved pregabalin 75 mg once daily in the evening for 3 days and then titrate up by 75 mg every 3 days up to 300 mg per day (150 mg morning and 150 mg evening).

This patient was started on pregabalin up to 300 mg per day. His pain was slightly improved (15–20%) and he slept better, but he reported dizziness, fatigue, and somnolence. Thus, you may downgrade pregabalin gradually (by steps of 75 mg every 3 days) and introduce gabapentin, which is sometimes better tolerated: 300 mg in the evening and then titrate up by steps of 300 mg every 3 days up to 1800 mg per day (maximal dosage 3600 mg/day). The patient tolerated gabapentin 1800 mg well and reported 60% reduction of pain.

Another option would be to stop fluoxetine gradually and introduce duloxetine (which has antidepressant effects at similar dosages) to maintain drugs as monotherapy. You may start with duloxetine 30 mg per day during meal (to reduce the risk of nausea) and then 60 mg daily after 1 week (BID or once daily). You should not combine duloxetine and fluoxetine because both are effective at relatively high dosages (there is a potential risk of serotonin syndrome).

If response is insufficient with the first drug (<30% pain relief), you may switch to another drug (this means that you have to taper off the first drug progressively while increasing the second) or combine drug classes to enhance or restore efficacy. In a large-scale trial, it was found that patients unresponsive to monotherapy with duloxetine 60 mg or pregabalin 300 mg were responders again if they increased dosages (to 120 mg and 600 mg, respectively) or combined duloxetine and pregabalin at the same dosages, with no

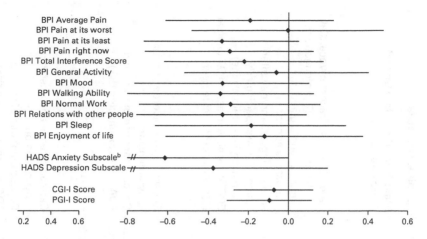

FIGURE 27.1 Effects of the combination of moderate dosages of duloxetine (60 mg/day) and pregabalin (300 mg/day) over monotherapy at high dosages (120 mg and 600 mg daily for duloxetine and pregabalin, respectively) in patients with diabetic painful neuropathy who did not respond to monotherapy at moderate dosages (the COMBO-DN study; Tesfaye et al., 2013). There was no significant difference on the primary outcome (not shown), but many secondary outcomes favored the combination. This suggests that it is relevant to combine these drugs to achieve better global efficacy in patients who do not respond to monotherapy at moderate dosages. BPI, Brief Pain Inventory; CGI-I, Clinical Global Impression of Improvement; HADS, Hospital Anxiety and Depression Scale; PGI-I, Patient Global Impression of Improvement.

risk of further side effects (Figure 27.1). It is not recommended to combine pregabalin and gabapentin (same mechanisms of action) or antidepressants and tramadol (potential risk of serotonin syndrome, because tramadol, an opioid agonist, also acts on the reuptake of serotonin). In case of efficacy (at least 50% pain relief), it is necessary to maintain drugs for at least 6 months and then taper them off gradually and try to stop them.

The mainstay of therapy for neuropathic pain includes antidepressants and antiepileptics, but not all have the same efficacy.

Antidepressants effective for neuropathic pain and generally recommended first line include tricyclic antidepressants (amitriptyline, clomipramine, imipramine, nortriptyline, and desipramine: 10–150 mg/day, average 25–75 mg/day) and serotonin–norepinephrine reuptake inhibitors (SNRIs) duloxetine (60–120 mg/day) and venlafaxine (150–225 mg/day). They have specific analgesic effects (by acting mainly on descending modulatory controls): Their analgesic effects are independent on their antidepressant effects, and their

TABLE 27.1   Antidepressants and Antiepileptics Recommended for Neuropathic Pain or Trigeminal Neuralgia

Drugs and Dosages	Official Approval for Use	Adverse Effects	Main Precautions for Use and Contraindications
Tricyclic antidepressants			
Amitriptyline, clomipramine, imipramine, nortriptyline, desipramine 10–75 mg (max. 150 mg) once daily or in 2 divided doses	FDA: no approval for use in analgesia EMA: approved in select countries for neuropathic pain	Somnolence, confusion (less nortriptyline/ desipramine), sweating, dry mouth, dysuria, constipation, weight gain, sexual effects (impotence, reduced libido), hyponatremia, hepatitis, seizures	Cardiac disease (recent myocardial infarction and QT prolongation), narrow angle glaucoma, prostatic adenoma Avoid using ≥75 mg/day after age 65 years (particularly amitriptyline, imipramine) ECG at baseline to assess QT interval FDA blackbox (suicide risk)
Serotonin–norepinephrine reuptake inhibitors			
Duloxetine 30–120 mg once daily or in 2 divided doses	FDA: diabetic painful neuropathy and chronic musculoskeletal pain EMA: diabetic painful neuropathy	Nausea, abdominal pain, constipation, insomnia, sexual effects, increased liver enzymes, hyponatrema Many drug–drug interactions (e.g., warfarin)	Severe hepatic disorder, unstable hypertension Concomitant use of tramadol FDA blackbox (suicide risk)
Venlafaxine 75–225 mg once daily or in 2 divided doses	No approval in analgesia	Nausea, hypertension (dosages ≥225 mg per day), sexual effects, hyponatrema, increased liver enzymes	Cardiac disease and unstable hypertension Concomitant use of tramadol FDA blackbox (suicide risk)

Antiepileptics

Gabapentin 1200–3600 mg per day in 3 divided doses	FDA: diabetic painful neuropathy, postherpetic neuralgia EMA: peripheral neuropathic pain	Somnolence, dizziness, peripheral edema, weight gain Abuse reported	Reduce dose in renal insufficiency Contraindicated in severe renal insufficiency (creatinine clearance <30 ml/mn) Abuse potential
Pregabalin 150–600 mg per day in 2 or 3 divided doses	FDA: diabetic painful neuropathy, postherpetic neuralgia, spinal cord injury EMA: peripheral and central neuropathic pain	Same as for gabapentin	Same as for gabapentin
Carbamazepine 200–1200 mg per day in 2 divided doses	FDA/EMA: trigeminal neuralgia	Somnolence, dizziness, confusion, idiosyncratic effects (cutaneous rash, Lyell or Stevens–Johnson, hepatitis, hyponatremia, neutropenia), drug–drug interactions (++ oral contraceptives)	Contraindication if atrioventricular block ECG recommended at baseline Complete cell blood count (AST, ALT, ALP, GGT, sodium) at baseline then regular intervals
Oxcarbazepine 150–1200 mg per day in 2 divided doses	No approval in analgesia Recommended for trigeminal neuralgia	Same as for carbamazepine but less common except hyponatremia	Contraindication if atrioventricular block ECG recommended at baseline Complete cell blood count (AST, ALT, ALP, GGT, sodium) at baseline then regular intervals

ECG, electrocardiomyography; EMA, European Medicines Agency; FDA, U.S. Food and Drug Administration.

efficacy is similar in depressed and not depressed patients. In contrast, selective serotonin reuptake inhibitors (fluoxetine, paroxetine, citalopram, escitalopram, and sertraline) and other antidepressants (mianserin, mirtazapine, etc.) have poor analgesic effects (Table 27.1).

The antiepileptics gabapentin (1200–3600 mg daily) and pregabalin (150–600 mg daily) are effective for neuropathic pain and also generally recommended as first line. They have central mechanisms of action (by binding to a subunit of calcium channels, the $\alpha_2\delta$ subunit). The sodium channel blockers carbamazepine (600–1200 mg per day) and oxcarbazepine (900–2400 mg per day) are recommended for trigeminal neuralgia. Other antiepileptics (lamotrigine, lacosamide, and topiramate) have less established efficacy (and no approval for use in analgesia) (see Table 27.1).

KEY POINTS TO REMEMBER

- Antidepressants and antiepileptics are the mainstay of therapy for peripheral or central neuropathic pain, and their efficacy is independent of their antidepressant effects (for antidepressants) or their effects on seizures (for antiepileptics).
- SNRIs (duloxetine) and tricyclic antidepressants (amitriptyline and nortriptyline) are generally recommended as first line. They should not be combined.
- The antiepileptics pregabalin and gabapentin are generally recommended as first line with caution because of potential abuse. They should not be combined.
- The antiepileptics carbamazepine and oxcarbazepine are recommended for trigeminal neuralgia only.
- Antidepressants and antiepileptics may be combined at moderate dosages to optimize their efficacy without increasing side effects.

Further Reading

Attal N, Bouhassira D. Advances in the treatment of neuropathic pain. *Curr Opin Neurol.* 2021;34(5):631–637.

Colloca L, Ludman T, Bouhassira D, et al. Neuropathic pain. *Nat Rev Dis Primers.* 2017;3:17002.

Finnerup NB, Attal N, Haroutounian S, et al. Pharmacotherapy for neuropathic pain in adults: A systematic review and meta-analysis. *Lancet Neurol.* 2015;14(2):162–173.

Gilron I, Jensen TS, Dickenson AH. Combination pharmacotherapy for management of chronic pain: From bench to bedside. *Lancet Neurol.* 2013;12(11):1084–1095.

Moisset X, Bouhassira D, Avez Couturier J, et al. Pharmacological and non-pharmacological treatments for neuropathic pain: Systematic review and French recommendations. *Rev Neurol.* 2020;176(5):325–352.

Tesfaye S, Wilhelm S, Lledo A, et al. Duloxetine and pregabalin: High-dose monotherapy or their combination? The "COMBO-DN study" —a multinational, randomized, double-blind, parallel-group study in patients with diabetic peripheral neuropathic pain. *Pain.* 2013;154:2616–2625.

Nadine Attal and Didier Bouhassira

An 88-year-old woman suffers from postherpetic neuralgia with a well-circumscribed and limited area of pain under the breast, corresponding to the T6 left thoracic dermatome. She reports intense burning pain, itch, electric shocks, and evoked pain, which is so severe that she cannot use bras. She has been treated with gabapentin and duloxetine, but these drugs have induced too many side effects and have both been stopped. She is desperate to find any safe and easy-to-use drug therapy to alleviate her pain. Clinical examination reveals severe allodynia to brush and no evidence for sensory deficit in the painful area.

What do you do now?

This elderly woman with postherpetic neuralgia did not tolerate most of the first-line oral treatments for neuropathic pain, such as duloxetine or gabapentin. Rather than trying another oral drug therapy such as a tricyclic antidepressant (amitriptyline and nortriptyline) or pregabalin, it is advisable to propose a topical treatment for her pain. Other reasons for this choice are the fact that she has a well-circumscribed and limited area of pain, making it easy to use topical medications. Finally, she suffers from severe allodynia to brush and has no apparent sensory deficit, suggesting that nociceptive fibers are hyperexcitable and play a predominant role in her pain. This implies that topical agents, which mainly act on peripheral mechanisms, should have some efficacy. Conversely, topical agents are expected to have less efficacy if the pain is present in an area of total sensory loss.

Topical agents investigated in peripheral neuropathic pain (i.e., postherpetic neuralgia, painful neuropathies, and painful post-traumatic/postsurgical nerve lesions) mainly include lidocaine 5% plasters (second line; U.S. Food and Drug Administration [FDA] and European Medicines Agency [EMA] approval for postherpetic neuralgia) in primary care Figures 28.1), and, for specialized setting, capsaicin high-concentration patches (FDA approval for postherpetic neuralgia and diabetic peripheral neuropathy of the feet; EMA approval for peripheral neuropathic

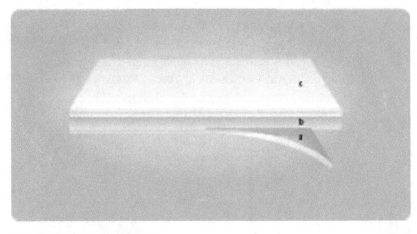

FIGURE 28.1 5% lidocaine plasters.

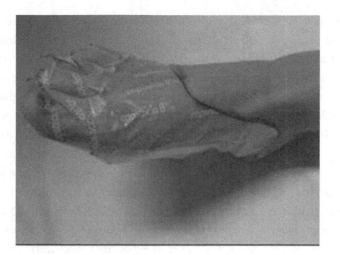

FIGURE 28.2 Capsaicin high-concentration patches applied to the foot for a patient with painful neuropathy.

pain in adults) and botulinum toxin A (off label in neuropathic pain) (Figures 28.2, 28.3).

This woman was initially treated by lidocaine 5% plasters (three plasters for 12 consecutive hours every day) with partial efficacy on burning pain and electric shocks (20%). Given this modest efficacy, capsaicin high-concentration patches were proposed in specialist settings: one and a half

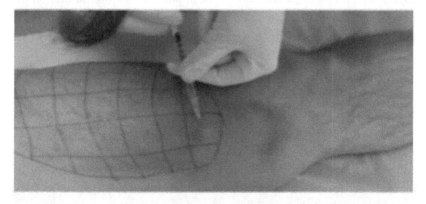

FIGURE 28.3 Photograph showing the injection process for botulinum toxin A in a patient with post-traumatic neuropathic pain.

patches were applied on the painful area during 60 minutes. However, she reported severe side effects (redness, edema, and burning) that lasted for more than 7 days and were only partially alleviated by cold application and acetaminophen 3 g per day. She states that she does not wish to try capsaicin patches again. Hence, she was referred to a specialist who proposed to treat her pain with subcutaneous botulinum toxin A. He injected 100 units subcutaneously in her painful area (5 units per cm^2). After 7 days, she started to feel significant pain relief: Relief was marked on paroxysmal pain (40%) and allodynia (30%). Since then, she has applied lidocaine plasters every day and receives botulinum toxin injections every 3 months. After 1 year, her pain intensity has been reduced by 50%. She is now able to resume her everyday activity. This case report illustrates that it is possible to combine several topical agents due to their distinct mechanisms and their different modalities of applications.

Lidocaine plasters act on neuronal hyperexcitability through sodium channel-blocking properties. Their efficacy has been established mainly in postherpetic neuralgia. Up to three patches can be applied to intact skin for 12 hours per day. Side effects are mainly local with skin irritation or allergy.

Capsaicin activates transient receptor potential vanilloid 1 ligand-gated channels on nociceptive fibers, subsequently leading to desensitization and defunctionalization of nociceptive fibers. The sustained efficacy (for about 3 months) of high-concentration capsaicin patches (8%) has been confirmed in postherpetic neuralgia, and diabetic and HIV painful neuropathies. Up to four patches have to be applied for 30–60 minutes on the painful area. Side effects are mainly skin reactions with redness, pain, and itching for up to a few days after application. The long-term safety of repeated applications seems favorable.

Botulinum toxin A, a potent neurotoxin used for the treatment of focal muscle hyperactivity, has shown efficacy in neuropathic pain for up to 3 months after a single set of injections (the administrations are conducted intradermally or subcutaneously in the painful area). One multicenter trial indicated the efficacy of repeated administrations over 6 months, with enhanced effects of the second injection. Doses range from 100 to 400 IU divided over the area of pain. Since the application may be painful, local anesthetics and inhalation of 50% nitrous oxide and oxygen can be used before and throughout the treatment to minimize the pain.

KEY POINTS TO REMEMBER

- Lidocaine plasters 5% (one to three plasters per day adapted to the painful area) and high-concentration capsaicin patches (one to four patches every 3 months adapted to the painful area, specialized setting) are recommended, for peripheral neuropathic pain with local pain generator (e.g., painful nerve lesion, painful neuropathies, and postherpetic neuralgia).
- Botulinum toxin A (subcutaneous or intradermal injection of 50–300 units every 3 months adapted to the painful area) is also recommended by specialist use but has no approval for use.

Further Reading

Attal N, Bouhassira D. Advances in the treatment of neuropathic pain. *Curr Opin Neurol.* 2021;34(5):631–637.

Attal N, de Andrade DC, Adam F, et al. Safety and efficacy of repeated injections of botulinum toxin A in peripheral neuropathic pain (BOTNEP): A randomised, double-blind, placebo-controlled trial. *Lancet Neurol.* 2016;15(6):555–565.

Colloca L, Ludman T, Bouhassira D, et al. Neuropathic pain. *Nat Rev Dis Primers.* 2017;3:17002.

Finnerup NB, Attal N, Haroutounian S, et al. Pharmacotherapy for neuropathic pain in adults: A systematic review and meta-analysis. *Lancet Neurol.* 2015;14(2):162–173.

Moisset X, Bouhassira D, Avez Couturier J, et al. Pharmacological and non-pharmacological treatments for neuropathic pain: Systematic review and French recommendations. *Rev Neurol.* 2020;176(5):325–352.

Pickering G, Voute M, Macian N, Ganry H, Pereira B. Effectiveness and safety of 5% lidocaine-medicated plaster on localized neuropathic pain after knee surgery: A randomized, double-blind controlled trial. *Pain.* 2019;160:1186–1195.

29 Opioids

Michael C. Rowbotham

A 38-year-old man was injured on the job 3 years ago
and has undergone two operations on his lumbar
spine. Recent magnetic resonance imaging shows no
operable lesions, and electromyography and nerve
conduction tests show unilateral radiculopathy (L4,
L5, and S1). He has not returned to full-time work.
He continues to receive short-term disability via a
worker's compensation program and has applied
for permanent disability status. He was placed on
opioids soon after the injury and continues daily use
of oxycodone 30 mg twice daily plus hydromorphone
4 mg for breakthrough pain (twice daily). Duloxetine
was stopped due to nausea. Four epidural steroid
injections failed to reduce pain . During his early 20s,
he was treated for alcohol abuse and had one arrest
for driving under the influence; he and one sibling had
frequent cocaine/amphetamine use into their early 30s
without legal consequences. He rates his pain as 7/10
every day, with peaks of 9/10.

What do you do now?

This man suffering from chronic low back pain with a neuropathic component has multiple "red flags" for developing problematic opioid use. He has a prior history of cocaine/amphetamine use and alcohol abuse. His current regimen consists entirely of short-acting opioids. He was placed on opioids soon after his injury, remains on disability, and has not successfully returned to work. You need to know more about his psychological profile (this may require a psychological or psychiatrist advice) and support (whether he is receiving counseling services or belongs to a support group). You should also search for other potential complicating factors, such as ongoing litigation, psychological issues (depression and family dysfunction), relapse to alcohol abuse, potential signs of opioid withdrawal, and use of illegal opioids or selling prescribed opioids (this was not the case here). This patient may be considered as having opioid use disorder (OUD) because of his high daily doses (the higher the daily opioid doses, the higher the risk; this generally occurs for doses higher than 120 mg morphine equivalent per day), but he has only mild withdrawal symptoms (these might account for times when his pain is 9/10) and tolerance to morphine (which starts relatively quickly after opioid initiation). His OUD remains mild (Box 29.1).

You now need to examine his opioid regimen in detail. He is taking two different opioids, both immediate-release oxycodone and hydromorphone. These opioids have a short duration of action (approximately 2–6 hours when used long term, and end-of-dose phenomena may include worsening pain and symptoms of withdrawal). Adding a short-acting to a long-acting opioid to serve as a rescue for "breakthrough" pain (which, in the case of neuropathic pain, generally corresponds to paroxysmal pain such as electric shocks) carries significant risks. If he takes the "breakthrough" medication every day, especially several times a day, it is no longer an as-needed opioid but, rather, part of the overall regimen. Therefore, long-term use of regular short-acting opioids for non-cancer pain, including neuropathic pain, is not recommended.

You may envisage a progressive opioid dose reduction and even discontinuation (this may be beneficial in such patients) while initiating other recommended treatments because he has not had first- or second-line medications for neuropathic pain other than duloxetine (e.g., tricyclic antidepressants, gabapentin, pregabalin, physical therapy, and has

BOX 29.1 Diagnostic Criteria for Opioid Use Disorder

Check all that apply:

____ Opioids are often taken in larger amounts or over a longer period of time than intended.

____ There is a persistent desire or unsuccessful efforts to cut down or control opioid use.

____ A great deal of time is spent in activities necessary to obtain the opioid, use the opioid, or recover from its effects.

____ Recurrent opioid use resulting in failure to fulfill major role obligations at work, school, or home.

____ Important social, occupational, or recreational activities are given up or reduced because of opioid use.

____ Craving, or a strong desire to use opioids.

____ Continued opioid use despite having persistent or recurrent social or interpersonal problems caused or exacerbated by the effects of opioids.

____ Recurrent opioid use in situations in which it is physically hazardous.

____ Continued use despite knowledge of having a persistent or recurrent physical or psychological problem that is likely to have been caused or exacerbated by opioids.

____ Tolerance, as defined by *either* of the following:

    (a) A need for markedly increased amounts of opioids to achieve intoxication or desired effect.

    (b) Markedly diminished effect with continued use of the same amount of an opioid.

____ Withdrawal, as manifested by *either* of the following:

    (a) The characteristic opioid withdrawal syndrome.

    (b) The same (or a closely related) substance are taken to relieve or avoid withdrawal symptoms.

Total number of boxes checked: _____
Severity: mild, 2–3 symptoms; moderate, 4–5 symptoms; severe, 6 or more symptoms.

Source: American Psychiatric Association. *Diagnostic and Statistical Manual of Mental Disorders*. 5th ed. Washington, DC: American Psychiatric Association; 2013:541.

not tried transcutaneous electrical nerve stimulation, which may be appropriate in this context). However, this is not a unilateral decision by the physician, and he may be extremely anxious about the risk of uncontrollable pain during tapering. You need to agree with him on the need for taper, the target (complete or partial), rate, and how he may contact you during the taper to manage the inevitable bumps and setbacks. If he agrees to taper off opioids, it is preferable to estimate his morphine milligram equivalents (MME) or morphine equivalent doses, which is the potency of an opioid dose relative to morphine. You may use a conversion table (although conversions are approximate because individuals may respond differently to various opioids and tables are not based on large-scale studies). The daily morphine equivalents of the rescue opioid are added to those of the long-acting drug, and the total daily MME may be higher than expected. This patient receives oral oxycodone 30 mg twice daily plus hydromorphone 4 mg for breakthrough pain (usually twice per day). The total MME is 152 mg per day (60 × 2 for oxycodone and 8 × 4 for hydromorphone). It is advised to switch oxycodone and hydromorphone to one single oral short-lasting opioid, such as oral morphine, every 4–6 hours at fixed schedules and not for potential breakthrough (e.g., 140 mg morphine in four divided doses of 30–40 mg), and then continue to remove 10 mg each week. A complete taper may be difficult, but long-term maintenance at low doses under close supervision can be successful with a favorable risk:benefit ratio. This may be done concomitantly with a second trial of oral duloxetine, this time starting from low dosages (30 mg per day) during meal to decrease the risk of nausea (you may add an anti-nausea treatment for a few days). You may also need alprazolam 0.25 mg or another benzodiazepine for potential anxiety.

Another option would be to simplify his regimen to a single long-acting opioid, which may reduce withdrawal-related pain. Then you may start with a lower dose of the long-acting opioid than suggested by the equivalence table (e.g., sustained-release morphine 60 mg every 12 hours), warning him that dose adjustment might be necessary, and continuing for a short period a much lower dose of the short-acting opioid in order to discontinue it. Even if you choose this option, you would need to combine his sustained-release opioid with an antineuropathic drug and attempt discontinuation of opioids later, if possible.

TABLE 29.1 **Opioids Recommended for Neuropathic Pain in Adults**

Drug, Dosages, and Official Approval for Use in Analgesia	Mechanism of Action	Adverse Effects	Main Precautions for Use and Contraindications
Second line			
Tramadol (SR) 200–400 mg BID FDA/EMA: moderate/ severe pain	Mu receptor agonist and monoamine reuptake inhibition	Nausea, vomiting, constipation, dizziness, somnolence, abuse, seizures	History of substance abuse, suicide risk, use of antidepressants (particularly high dosages), patients aged ≥75 years (confusion), unstable seizures
Third line			
SR morphine, oxycodone Individual titration FDA/EMA approval for refractory pain, particularly cancer	Mu receptor agonists Oxycodone may also cause κ-receptor antagonism	Nausea, vomiting, constipation, dizziness, confusion, respiratory depression, pruritus, somnolence, dysuria, abuse	History of substance abuse, suicide risk, risk of misuse on long-term use Avoid ≥140 mg equivalent morphine in primary care

EMA, European Medicines Agency; FDA, U.S. Food and Drug Administration; SR, sustained release.

Contrary to preconceptions, strong opioids are more effective in peripheral chronic neuropathic pain than in back pain and other pains exacerbated by physical movement, such as osteoarthritis (results are also poor in central pain and complex regional pain syndrome). However, they are only recommended as third line for neuropathic pain (Table 29.1). Those with best established efficacy include sustained-release oral morphine and oxycodone, but transdermal fentanyl and oral methadone may also be considered; doses have to be achieved by individual titration and kept at low to moderate dosages, corresponding to <140 mg per day of morphine equivalent. Sustained-release tramadol (100–400 mg per day), a weak opioid with additional effects on monoamine reuptake, is recommended as second line for neuropathic pain, but it may have similar potential abuse risks as strong opioids, depending on the doses (Table 29.1). Weak opioids (codeine and dihydrocodeine) are poorly effective.

When a physician prescribes opioids for a patient, an agreement should be set for monitoring and potential consequences if the agreement is violated. Like in a methadone maintenance program, there should be only one opioid prescriber who controls doses and types of opioid, manages prescription refills, works with other clinicians to set goals, and ensures that corrective action (even opioid tapering or discontinuation) is taken if the patient does not adhere to mutually agreed-upon guidelines. Early warning signs of OUD should lead to more frequent contact, reduction of pills, and no automatic prescription refills. Urine monitoring has a role, and if OUD seems likely, referral to a specialized program (even hospitalization in some cases) is warranted.

KEY POINTS TO REMEMBER

- Red flags for problematic opioid use include current or past alcohol, stimulant, or sedative abuse; frequent requests for dose escalation or doses above 120 MEQ/day; and criteria for OUD or addiction.
- Much like patients in a methadone maintenance program, there should be only one opioid prescriber who controls dose and type of opioid and manages frequency of prescription refills.

- Opioids are not a first-line therapy for chronic pain (they are generally recommended as second line for tramadol and as third line for strong opioids). Prior trials of antidepressants (tricyclic antidepressants and serotonin–norepinephrine reuptake inhibitors), gabapentinoids, and neuromodulation should be well documented.
- The most difficult part of tapering off opioids for patients is anxiety and fear of uncontrollable pain. A complete taper may be unrealistic, but long-term maintenance at low doses under close supervision can be successful with a favorable risk:benefit ratio.
- Opioid analgesic tolerance starts relatively quickly after opioids are initiated, but opioid-induced hyperalgesia is not yet proven to be a common clinically relevant phenomenon.

Further Reading

Calculating total daily dose of opioids for safer dosage. Centers for Disease Control and Prevention. https://www.cdc.gov/drugoverdose/pdf/calculating_total_daily_dose-a.pdf

Finnerup NB, Attal N, Haroutounian S, et al. Pharmacotherapy for neuropathic pain in adults: A systematic review and meta-analysis. *Lancet Neurol*. 2015;14(2):162–173.

Opioid conversion table. American Academy of Family Physicians. https://www.aafp.org/dam/AAFP/documents/patient_care/pain_management/conversion-table.pdf

Opioid use disorder: What is opioid addition? Providers Clinical Support System. https://pcssnow.org/resource/opioid-use-disorder-opioid-addiction

30 Physical Therapy

Nadine Attal, Grégory Tosti, and Didier Bouhassira

A 42-year-old right-handed woman suffers from chronic pain of the right hand after surgery for carpal tunnel syndrome 1 year ago. She reports burning pain of the hand extending to the forearm and arm. Pain is evoked by movement, touch, and cold, such that she now only uses her left hand for everyday activities. She also complains of tingling and numbness of the hand. At inspection, she has a guarding position of the painful hand, which is enveloped in a compression bandage. Clinical examination discloses edema of the hand, sudomotor changes, hypoalgesia to pinprick, and extreme allodynia to brush, pressure, and thermal stimuli, without apparent motor deficit, although this is difficult to ascertain because of the allodynia.

What do you do now?

This woman fulfills criteria for complex regional pain syndrome (CRPS) (see also Chapter 9). She dramatically underuses her hand, which is probably related to pain at movement but probably also to a hand neglect, as often reported in CRPS; this in turn increases her pain through a vicious circle.

Guidelines recommend the inclusion of physiotherapy as part of multi-modal management of CRPS, but this also applies to the management of any neuropathic pain syndrome. The best indications include motor deficit or neglect, major sensory deafferentation, physical deconditioning, and fear of pain and movement (as is often the case for low back pain with or without leg pain).

For this woman, you should prescribe physical therapy by a physiotherapist aiming to restore her hand range of motion. However, physical exercises may be initially very painful in case of CRPS, and this may have negative consequences on her recovery. Hence, you should prescribe a strong analgesic, such as oral nefopam or immediate-release strong opioids (oral morphine 10 mg) 1 hour before each exercise to facilitate rehabilitation. If pain is not relieved sufficiently by oral drugs, some patients may be referred to anesthesiologists for a temporary regional analgesic blockade to allow rehabilitation. After a few months of physical therapy, this woman partially recovered her range of motion, but severe pain is still present. More invasive therapeutic strategies, including spinal cord stimulation, are now being discussed.

Physiotherapy may be broadly defined as treatment with any physical agent and method and thus includes a large variety of interventions, particularly manual therapy; therapeutic exercises including physical reconditioning; electrotherapy (e.g., transcutaneous electrical nerve stimulation); and sensorimotor rehabilitation strategies, including mirror therapy and graded motor imagery (GMI). Immersive virtual reality (VR), which is a more recent approach, may also be considered in the spectrum of physical therapy techniques.

Therapeutic exercises and manual therapy (e.g., mobilization, manipulation, massages, and desensitization) may induce analgesia via endogenous opioid controls and improve function and disability by restoring range of movement and improving neuromuscular function. Randomized controlled trials have suggested that multimodal physiotherapy may be beneficial in reducing the pain and disability associated with CRPS and other neuropathic pains, particularly phantom limb pain and spinal cord injury pain, but the quality of evidence is considered to be low. Despite limited evidence, consensus-based recommendations support the use of multimodal rehabilitation as first-line therapy for CRPS.

Mirror therapy consists of concealing the painful limb behind a mirror and simultaneously moving the portion of the intact limb and painful limb (this generally corresponds to movement intention in patients with paraplegia or phantom limb) while observing the reflection of the intact limb in the mirror (Figure 30.1). This provides visual illusion that the movement intention of the painful limb is successful. GMI uses a graded sequence of strategies, including left/right judgments (this aims to distinguish a body part belonging to the left side from that of the right side of the body), imagined movements (imagining moving the limb into various postures), and mirror therapy. Both mirror therapy and GMI may provide pain relief

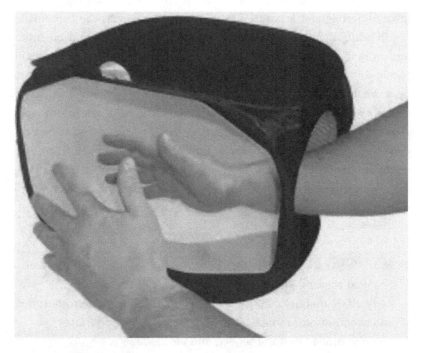

FIGURE 30.1 Mirror therapy.

by improving maladaptive somatosensory and motor cortex reorganization, and they have been combined with brain neurostimulation techniques such as transcranial direct current stimulation of the motor cortex to enhance efficacy in some trials. Best evidence for efficacy of these techniques stems from small positive studies of GMI and mirror therapy in CRPS, phantom limb pain, and central pain due to spinal cord injury, but negative results have also been published. The lack of standardization and homogeneity of these techniques in randomized trials renders interpretation of the results extremely difficult. Limb discomfort seems to be the most commonly identified adverse effect in studies of sensory motor rehabilitation strategies.

Virtual reality (VR) is a computer-generated environment that immerses the user in an interactive artificial world, thus allowing a detour of attention from external sensory afferents. Initial studies have highlighted the effectiveness of VR for acute pain. Underlying mechanisms probably involve a modification of the activity of the autonomic nervous system and a reduction in the activity of the brain regions involved in nociceptive processing, but other mechanisms seem common to the neurophysiological changes observed in conditioning and exposure therapies. In this context, the combination of VR with cognitive–behavioral therapy-type therapies could potentially lead to new treatment options for chronic pain. In the context of neuropathic pain, particularly CRPS, phantom pain, or spinal cord injury pain, neurorehabilitation techniques may use VR systems to restore movement and relieve the pain, thus recalling the works carried out by mirror therapy. However, analgesic effects vary from study to study, and the question of the persistence of analgesic effects arises, although in one recent small crossover randomized controlled trial, patients suggested a medium-term benefit in spinal cord injury pain. Thus, VR seems encouraging for the treatment of pain, but currently evidence mostly concerns the treatment of acute pain.

KEY POINTS TO REMEMBER

· Physical therapy includes a large variety of interventions, particularly manual therapy; therapeutic exercises; electrotherapy; and sensorimotor rehabilitation strategies, including mirror therapy, graded motor imagery, and virtual reality.

- Best evidence for the efficacy of physical therapy in neuropathic pain concerns mirror therapy and graded motor imagery (for CRPS and phantom limb pain), but there are very few studies supporting their long-term efficacy.
- Despite a paucity of well-designed studies, multimodal physical therapy is recommended as first line for CRPS based on expert consensus.
- Virtual reality is increasingly investigated for the treatment of acute pain, but there are limited data regarding its efficacy on neuropathic pain.

Further Reading

Austin PD, Craig A, Middleton JW, et al. The short-term effects of head-mounted virtual-reality on neuropathic pain intensity in people with spinal cord injury pain: A randomised cross-over pilot study. *Spinal Cord.* 2021;59:738–746.

Chuan A, Zhou JJ, Hou RM, Stevens CJ, Bogdanovych A. Virtual reality for acute and chronic pain management in adult patients: A narrative review. *Anaesthesia.* 2021;76:695–704.

Colloca L, Raghuraman N, Wang Y, et al. Virtual reality: Physiological and behavioral mechanisms to increase individual pain tolerance limits. *Pain.* 2020;161:2010–2021.

Smart KM, Wand BM, O'Connell NE. Physiotherapy for pain and disability in adults with complex regional pain syndrome (CRPS) types I and II. *Cochrane Database Syst Rev.* 2016;2:CD010853.

Thieme H, Morkisch N, Rietz C, Dohle C, Borgetto B. The efficacy of movement representation techniques for treatment of limb pain—A systematic review and meta-analysis. *J Pain.* 2016;17:167–180.

Xie HM, Zhang KX, Wang S, et al. Effectiveness of mirror therapy for phantom limb pain: A systematic review and meta-analysis. *Arch Phys Med Rehabil.* 2022;103(5):988–997.

31 Psychotherapies: How, When, and Why

Nadine Attal and Didier Bouhassira

A 49-year-old woman suffers from severe neuropathic pain (described as burning) after surgical intervention 3 years ago for right carpal tunnel syndrome. She is divorced and lives with her 15-year-old son who has intellectual disability, she is in work cessation (she was a bank employee) mainly because of moral harassment, and seldom leaves her home except to accompany her son to his day care program three times a week. She feels that the pain will never go away. She is afraid of moving her right arm, which she protects from movements with a self-made bandage. She receives amitriptyline and pregabalin, with very weak efficacy on her pain, and lorazepam for anxiety and sleep disorders, which she finds less effective over time. Examination discloses no motor deficit or reflex abnormalities, but sensory examination shows extended brush-evoked pain (involving the whole arm and trunk), and edema, skin redness, and sudation of the arm.

What do you do now?

This woman who underwent surgery for carpal tunnel syndrome is suffering considerably. She has experienced multiple life events (divorce, disabled child, and financial and work problems) and suffers from social isolation, which contribute to enhance her pain. The spread of evoked pain outside the neuroanatomical area of the lesioned nerve suggests central amplification and/or sensitization phenomena, probably enhanced by her anxiety. This suggests that her neuropathic pain coexists with nociplastic pain (regional chronic pain not entirely explained by the nerve lesion, with symptoms and signs of hypersensitivity spreading outside the neuroanatomical area of the nerve lesion and comorbidities).

This woman needs therapeutic education and counseling as a first step to better understand her pain and the nature of treatments. This may be conducted on an individual or group basis. In particular, she needs to understand that long-term immobilization of her hand resulted in increased pain, thus causing a vicious circle, and that long-term opioids are not an option. Then you should ask for psychological or psychiatric advice. Psychiatric assessment showed that this woman had panic attacks and many dysfunctional thoughts about her pain. Hence, this woman is a good candidate for psychotherapy, provided that she accepts the constraints and necessity to attend several therapeutic sessions.

This woman accepted a program of 10 sessions of cognitive-behavioral therapy (CBT), together with progressive physical reconditioning. After 6 months, her pain was only slightly improved (5/10), but she was able to resume most of her past everyday activities, see friends again, and stopped protecting her arm. Her quality of life and sleep improved partially. She now envisages to resume her professional activity in another position at the bank where she worked.

Psychological therapy plays a major role in the management of chronic neuropathic pain, as for other pain conditions. It aims to decrease dysfunctional coping strategies, thoughts about pain, and catastrophizing, which are common consequences of chronic pain, and improve anxiety and mood. Hence, it not only contributes to improve pain and mood but also may impact self-efficacy and return to work. CBT has been the most studied (Table 31.1). It may include role-playing, relaxation, and mental distractions, and it is generally administered by psychologists or psychiatrists.

TABLE 31.1 Main Principles of Cognitive–Behavioral Therapy and Acceptance and Commitment Therapy

Therapy	Principles in Adults
Cognitive–behavioral therapy	Typical protocols include the following: Cognitive appraisal of negative beliefs and thoughts about pain. Emotional regulation and exposure to reduce the anticipation of pain and avoid negative thoughts about pain. Behavioral engagement with rewarding activities. Skills in problem-solving and motivation.
Acceptance and commitment therapy	Acceptance and commitment therapy is an extension of cognitive–behavioral therapy, with a focus on flexibility in action, a willingness to experience pain without struggle, the recognition that thoughts are not facts but are open to interpretation, and the promotion of values-based action.

Adapted and modified from Williams et al. (2020).

Web-delivered CBT has also considerably expanded because of the COVID-19 pandemic. A recent Cochrane analysis of psychotherapies for chronic pain found evidence (based on 59 studies including more than 5,000 participants) that CBT has modest efficacy (with low to moderate quality of evidence) on pain, disability, and distress in chronic pain. Conditions encompassed fibromyalgia, chronic low back pain, rheumatoid arthritis, and multi-etiology chronic pain. However, evidence is weak with regard to neuropathic pain. Ideal candidates should be motivated and report maladaptive thoughts about their pain or mood/anxiety disorders, but the nature of neuropathic pain and its intensity and duration do not impact the efficacy of CBT (although very old age may be a limiting factor). In recent years, mindfulness (see Chapter 32) has been incorporated in psychotherapies, including mindfulness-based cognitive therapy—therapy based on mindfulness for the reduction of stress mindfulness-oriented recovery enhancement. Mindfulness is mainly focused on the present, trying to increase awareness and acceptance of the emotional and physical suffering.

- Among psychotherapies, CBT has been the most studied for chronic pain; there are very few studies of CBT specifically regarding neuropathic pain.
- Psychotherapies may be recommended as stand-alone or add-on to other treatments.
- Best candidates should be motivated and educated subjects, with maladaptive thoughts about their neuropathic pain and/or mood or anxiety disorders.

Further Reading

Cohen SP, Vase L, Hooten WM. Chronic pain: An update on burden, best practices, and new advances. *Lancet*. 2021;397:2082–2097.

Eccleston C, Blyth FM, Dear BF, et al. Managing patients with chronic pain during the COVID-19 outbreak: Considerations for the rapid introduction of remotely supported (eHealth) pain management services. *Pain*. 2020;161(5):889–893.

Knoerl R, Smith EML, Barton DL, et al. Self-guided online cognitive behavioral strategies for chemotherapy-induced peripheral neuropathy: A multicenter, pilot, randomized, wait-list controlled trial. *J Pain*. 2018;19:382–394.

Kosek E, Clauw D, Nijs J, Baron R, Gilron I, Harris RE, Mico JA, Rice ASC, Sterling M. Chronic nociplastic pain affecting the musculoskeletal system: clinical criteria and grading system. *Pain*. 2021;162:2629–2634.

Moisset X, Bouhassira D, Avez Couturier J, et al. Pharmacological and non-pharmacological treatments for neuropathic pain: Systematic review and French recommendations. *Rev Neurol*. 2020;176(5):325–352.

Williams ACC, Fisher E, Hearn L, Eccleston C. Psychological therapies for the management of chronic pain (excluding headache) in adults. *Cochrane Database Syst Rev*. 2020;8(8):CD007407.

32 Complementary Medicine

Grégory Tosti

A 74-year-old man has been suffering from alcoholic painful neuropathy for approximately 10 years. Pain is refractory to several lines of well-conducted drug treatments and to motor cortex repetitive transcranial magnetic stimulation. The patient does not wish to receive invasive therapy. Clinical interview and evaluation reveal severe pain intensity (numeric rating scale, 8/10), excessive focus on pain with catastrophizing, sleep disorders, and increasing difficulty coping with stressful situations. Given the refractory nature of the pain as well as the severity and its impact on his daily life (increased stress, difficulty in managing anxiety-provoking situations, sleep disorders, and fatigue), the patient was encouraged by his pain doctor to try hypnosis with a specialized practitioner.

What do you do now?

This patient is refractory to several lines of medications and has dysfunctional coping with excessive focus on his neuropathic pain. He was initially referred to a psychologist for cognitive–behavioral therapy but has difficulty complying with the exercises and even understanding the principles of therapy. Among several complementary techniques (hypnosis, mindfulness, and acupuncture), hypnosis may be proposed (Table 32.1). It is defined as a mode of psychological functioning by which a subject, in relation with a practitioner, experiences a modified state of consciousness allowing changes in perception.

Unless you have specific training in hypnosis, you may orient this patient to a trained caregiver (a medical doctor or a psychologist). There are very few contraindications (they mainly include ongoing psychosis). Side effects are very rare and concern transient anxiety, distress, or headache. Each hypnotic session usually includes an induction phase, in which the subject is asked to focus attention on objects (e.g., a light) or experiences (breathing or being in a favorite spot), followed by therapeutic suggestions aiming to alter pain perceptions, emotions, and dysfunctional thoughts about pain (Figure 32.1). The patient received 5 sessions of hypnosis by a medical doctor (the optimal number of sessions varies from 2 to 12 in clinical trials, with 8 being most common) and then was advised—as is generally recommended—to engage in home practice on a daily basis using audio recordings (self-hypnosis) to maintain positive effects. After 6 months, he became less focused on his pain and his pain intensity was alleviated by 30%, but he was not able to stop alcohol (this is not surprising because hypnotic analgesia does not use the same process as hypnosis for addictive behaviors). A consultation in addictology is now envisaged.

Although hypnosis has been shown to be effective for acute pain (mainly procedural pain), evidence is weak with regard to its effectiveness in chronic pain, particularly neuropathic pain, and most studies have concerned fibromyalgia, headache, and irritable bowel syndrome. Furthermore, whether hypnosis induces specific therapeutic effects compared to other psychological techniques has yet to be determined. Thus, in a recent randomized controlled study comparing several sessions of hypnotic analgesia (with self-hypnosis) to three other interventions (cognitive therapy using hypnosis to alter the meaning of pain, standard cognitive therapy, and pain education) in 174 patients with mainly low back pain (and some patients with

TABLE 32.1 Hypnosis, Mindfulness, and Acupuncture for Chronic Neuropathic Pain

Procedure	Definition	Evidence, Side Effects, and Contraindications	Proposed Mechanisms
Hypnosis	A mode of psychological functioning by which a subject, in relation with a practitioner, experiences a modified state of consciousness allowing changes in perception. May be practiced at home (self-hypnosis) and combined with relaxation or biofeedback.	Weak evidence for efficacy in nociplastic pain based on small RCTs. Virtually no side effects (transient anxiety or distress) and very few contraindications (active psychosis).	Modifications of activity in brain areas involved in sensory (somatosensory cortex) or emotion processing (anterior cingulate cortex) (fMRI), depending on whether hypnosis modulates pain intensity or unpleasantness.
Mindfulness	Focuses on increased awareness of one's body, emotions, and thoughts at the present time. Patients advised to actively practice at home.	Small RCTs have found efficacy (versus usual care or relaxation) in neuropathic pain. The highest quality study conducted in painful diabetic neuropathy showed effects on pain, quality of life, and catastrophizing. Virtually no side effects and very few contraindications (active psychosis).	Modifications in brain structures associated with pain perception, attention, and emotions (fMRI).
Acupuncture	Involves the insertion of fine needles into specific points on the body along virtual lines called meridians. The needling of these points is believed to rebalance the body's functioning and restore health.	Efficacy best established in musculoskeletal pain, headache, and osteoarthritis. Insufficient evidence in neuropathic pain but relevant if well circumscribed and associated with muscle pain. Rare side effects: local pain, bleeding, bruising, sometimes drowsiness, nausea, vagal syncope, or dizziness. Sepsis exceptional. Contraindications: coagulopathy, pregnancy, pacemaker (electroacupuncture).	Effects on endogenous opioids or diffuse noxious inhibitory controls.

fMRI, functional magnetic resonance imaging; RCT, randomized controlled trial.

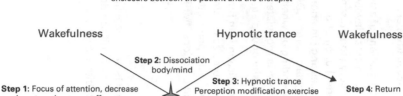

Modeling a hypnosis session

Experience of perceptual modification with a therapeutic aim taking place in the relational enclosure between the patient and the therapist

Wakefulness   Hypnotic trance   Wakefulness

Step 2: Dissociation
body/mind

Step 1: Focus of attention, decrease
in external sensory afferents

Step 3: Hypnotic trance
Perception modification exercise
(suggestions, mental imagery,
metaphors...)

Step 4: Return

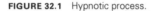

FIGURE 32.1 Hypnotic process.

Adapted from *L'hypnose Médicale*, 2nd ed. dir JM Benhaiem. MEDLINE; 2012.

neuropathic pain), all treatments were associated with similar improvements in pain intensity for up to 12 months after the end of sessions.

Other complementary techniques used for neuropathic pain patients include mindfulness, which may be effective based on randomized controlled trials, and acupuncture (see Table 32.1), but also relaxation, yoga, and biofeedback. The latter is a technique used to control stress through the body's functions, such as heart rate; during biofeedback, patients are connected to electrical sensors that help them receive information about their stress level.

> **KEY POINTS TO REMEMBER**
>
> · Hypnosis, mindfulness, and acupuncture may be proposed to patients with neuropathic pain, particularly as an add-on to conventional medications.
> · The level of evidence for their efficacy, specifically with regard to neuropathic pain, is limited and better documented for mindfulness.
> · There are no known predictors of the response to these treatments.

Further Reading

Derbyshire SW, Whalley MG, Oakley DA. Fibromyalgia pain and its modulation by hypnotic and non-hypnotic suggestion: An fMRI analysis. *Eur J Pain.* 2009;13(5):542–550.

Jensen MP, Day MA, Miró J. Neuromodulatory treatments for chronic pain: Efficacy and mechanisms. *Nat Rev Neurol.* 2014;10(3):167–178.

Jensen MP, Mendoza ME, Ehde D, et al. Effects of hypnosis, cognitive therapy, hypnotic cognitive therapy, and pain education in adults with chronic pain: A randomized clinical trial. *Pain* 2020;161(10):2284–2298.

Ju ZY, Wang K, Cui HS, et al. Acupuncture for neuropathic pain in adults. *Cochrane Database Syst Rev.* 2017;12(12):CD012057.

Kabat-Zinn, J. *Full Catastrophe Living: How to Cope with Stress, Pain and Illness Using Mindfulness Meditation.* Rev ed. Hachette; 2013.

Moisset X, Bouhassira D, Avez Couturier J, et al. Pharmacological and non-pharmacological treatments for neuropathic pain: Systematic review and French recommendations. *Rev Neurol.* 2020;176(5):325–352.

Nathan HJ, Poulin P, Wozny D, et al. Randomized trial of the effect of mindfulness-based stress reduction on pain-related disability, pain intensity, health-related quality of life, and A1C in patients with painful diabetic peripheral neuropathy. *Clin Diabetes.* 2017;35(5):294–304.

Yin C, Buchheit TE, Park JJ. Acupuncture for chronic pain: An update and critical overview. *Curr Opin Anaesthesiol.* 2017;30(5):583–592.

Zhang D, Lee EKP, Mak ECW, Ho CY, Wong SYS. Mindfulness-based interventions: An overall review. *Br Med Bull.* 2021;138(1):41–57.

33 Transcutaneous Electrical Nerve Stimulation

Nadine Attal and Didier Bouhassira

A 53-year-old active lawyer suffers from chronic left L5 sciatica despite surgery for discal herniation (failed back surgery syndrome) 1 year ago. Pain is described as burning, squeezing, and sometimes associated with electric shocks. It is not present at night and is moderate in the morning, but it tends to worsen in the evening when he returns home with an intensity of 6 or 7/10. There is no motor deficit, and tendon reflexes are normal. Sensory examination shows hypoesthesia to pinprick and cold in the painful area. Because of the necessity to maintain intellectual activity, he does not wish to take any oral medications for his pain. He has tried gabapentin, but this drug was stopped because of somnolence. Codeine–paracetamol and tramadol–paracetamol combinations caused attention disorders, and he was afraid of becoming dependent. Acetaminophen, ibuprofen, and lidocaine plasters were ineffective. He seeks a convenient treatment compatible with his professional activity.

What do you do now?

This patient has chronic peripheral neuropathic pain limited to the territory of the sciatic nerve (pain is well circumscribed). He has not tolerated oral medications and is reluctant to receive other drug therapies because of potentially disturbing side effects. He is a very good candidate for transcutaneous electrical nerve stimulation (TENS).

A TENS machine (several available models) is a small, battery-operated device with leads connected to sticky pads called electrodes (Figure 33.1). The pads are attached directly to the skin. When the machine is switched on, small electrical impulses are delivered to the affected area, which patients generally feel as paresthesia (tingling). Tolerability is excellent, with only minor skin irritations. There are virtually no contraindications except for pacemakers (TENS should then be avoided in the thoracic area).

TENS was prescribed to this patient for sessions of 30–60 minutes every evening. Modalities of use are variable (frequency from 0.5 to 120 Hz and intensity of stimulation up to 100 mA), and most machines have several programs with predetermined intensities and frequencies of stimulation. These modalities were determined during a training session with a specialized nurse before initiating therapy. He reported excellent efficacy (70%) after 15 minutes of use of TENS (predetermined frequency of stimulation 80 Hz and intensity of 50 mA) with an approximately 2-hour remanent effect, which corresponds to usual reporting in neuropathic pain.

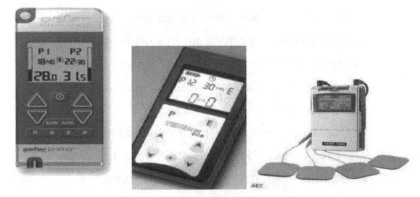

FIGURE 33.1 Example of TENS devices and electrodes.

TENS was introduced soon after Wall and Melzack conceived the largely disseminated gate control theory of pain in 1965, which proposed for the first time that the activity of large myelinated fibers was able to inhibit nociceptive input at the dorsal horn level. It is now established that mechanisms are not solely specifically related to effects on large fibers but also involve endogenous opioids and GABAergic inhibitory systems. TENS is slightly superior to placebo for peripheral neuropathic pain, including sciatica and painful neuropathies (low quality of evidence), whereas it is poorly effective on low back pain without radicular pain. TENS is recommended for peripheral neuropathic pain and has European Medicines Agency and U.S. Food and Drug Administration approval for use in analgesia.

Of note, TENS may also be used for pain through noninvasive vagal nerve stimulation. This may be achieved by placing an electrode on the ear to stimulate the tragus nerve, which contains approximately 1% of the vagus fibers. Transcutaneous vagus nerve stimulation may be a noninvasive alternative to invasive vagus nerve stimulation with implantable devices; it has been used mainly to treat drug-resistant epilepsy and depression. Efferents from the vagal nuclei receive sensory and visceral input and mainly course toward parts of the neural pain matrix via other vagal nuclei. Promising results of this technique have been observed in migraine, but there are no specific studies thus far in neuropathic pain.

KEY POINTS TO REMEMBER

- The efficacy of TENS is more established in neuropathic pain than in other types of pain, although the level of evidence remains weak.
- TENS may be recommended as stand-alone therapy or an add-on to other treatments.
- Safety and tolerability are excellent.
- Ideal candidates should have well-circumscribed peripheral neuropathic pain; best indications are chronic painful radiculopathy, some painful neuropathies (when the area of pain is limited), and post-traumatic/postsurgical nerve lesions.

Further Reading

Buchmuller A, Navez M, Milletre-Bernardin M, et al.; Lombotens Trial Group. Value of TENS for relief of chronic low back pain with or without radicular pain. *Eur J Pain*. 2012;16(5):656–665.

Clark O, Mahjoub A, Osman N, Surmava AM, Jan S, Lagman-Bartolome AM. Non-invasive neuromodulation in the acute treatment of migraine: A systematic review and meta-analysis of randomized controlled trials. *Neurol Sci*. 2022;43(1):153–165.

Gibson W, Wand BM, Meads C, Catley MJ, O'Connell NE. Transcutaneous electrical nerve stimulation (TENS) for chronic pain—An overview of Cochrane Reviews. *Cochrane Database Syst Rev*. 2019;4(4):CD011890.

Gibson W, Wand BM, O'Connell NE. Transcutaneous electrical nerve stimulation (TENS) for neuropathic pain in adults. *Cochrane Database Syst Rev*. 2017;9(9):CD011976.

Knotkova H, Hamani C, Sivanesan E, et al. Neuromodulation for chronic pain. *Lancet*. 2021;397(10289):2111–2124.

Moisset X, Bouhassira D, Avez Couturier J, et al. Pharmacological and non-pharmacological treatments for neuropathic pain: Systematic review and French recommendations. *Rev Neurol*. 2020;176(5):325–352.

Specialized Assessment and Therapy

34 Management of High-Risk Patients

Nadine Attal and Didier Bouhassira

A 68-year-old overweight woman is scheduled for total knee arthroplasty for chronic severe knee osteoarthritis. She consults you because she is extremely anxious about the risks of surgery, reading all she can find on websites. She also has increasingly more difficulty falling asleep; she ruminates about her surgery; and her mood has been very poor, with loss of interest, discouragement, and frequent panic attacks for the past 2 months. In addition, she states that she has used paracetamol codeine every day (six to eight pills a day, seldom more) for more than 1 year for migraine; she now reports headache every day. She has no signs of craving, and she sometimes overuses opioids only because of her severe headache. Because of the COVID-19 pandemic, her surgery was delayed by 3 months.

What do you do now?

This woman has several risk factors for developing chronic (neuropathic) pain after surgery, including her young age, pre-existing chronic pain (headache), opioid use, anxiety, depression, and catastrophizing (Table 34.1).

You should explain to her that the fact that surgery has been delayed is good news because this will provide time to manage her anxiety, depression, and migraine, such that she will be operated on in the best possible conditions. You should first encourage her to see a psychologist or psychiatrist. You may also gradually taper off opioids, which contribute to cause chronic daily headache, without asking for a specialist's advice because she does not have signs of abuse or craving. You should initiate a prophylactic treatment for her migraine, such as the tricyclic antidepressant amitriptyline (European Medicines Agency [EMA] approved for neuropathic pain and prophylactic treatment of migraine), because she has no contraindications (e.g., narrow-angle glaucoma or recent myocardial infarction). You should start with 5–10 mg daily at night (with drops) and then increase by steps of 10 mg every 4–7 days. Efficacy is generally observed at dosages of 75 mg daily for headache, and at this dosage the drug may also relieve depression. Main side effects include somnolence, confusion, dry mouth, sweating, constipation, dysuria, orthostatic hypotension, cardiac conduction block, and weight gain. Once this treatment is initiated, you should advise her to remove one or two tablets of paracetamol codeine every 4–7 days.

This woman started amitriptyline 10 mg at night. She saw a psychiatrist, who added alprazolam 0.25 mg for her panic attacks and increased the dosages up to 75 mg daily (which she reached after 8 weeks). She was able to taper off four tablets of paracetamol codeine per day. Prior to surgery, she also underwent psychotherapy conducted by a psychologist. Several well-conducted trials have indeed established the benefit of perioperative psychotherapy to reduce the risk of acute or chronic postsurgical pain.

Surgery was undertaken after 3 months. A few days after surgery, she felt numbness and tingling in the knee, suggesting a nerve lesion (probably the infrapatellar branch of the saphenous nerve). Psychotherapy was resumed. After 4 weeks, moderate pain appeared (intensity 5/10), described as aching, burning, and stabbing and involving the anterior face of the knee. Sensory examination disclosed slightly reduced pinprick sensation in the painful area. Because the pain characteristics and the area of pain were

TABLE 34.1   Risk Factors Identified for Chronic Postsurgical Pain, Including Neuropathic Pain

Domain	Preoperative Factors	Intraoperative Factors	Postoperative Factors
Demographics	Age Gender	NA	NA
Genetic	Gene mutations	NA	NA
Psychosocial	Depression Psychological vulnerability Stress Anxiety Cognitive flexibility Catastrophizing Alexithymia[1]	NA	Depression Psychological vulnerability Stress Anxiety Catastrophizing
Pain	Chronic pain Opioid use Hyperalgesia (experimental pain) Decreased pain modulation	NA	Severe acute pain Pain trajectory Acute neuropathic pain Acute hyperalgesia
Surgery	NA	Type of surgery Nerve lesion Duration of surgery Large incision	Revision surgery
Clinical	Comorbidities Disability	NA	Radiotherapy Chemotherapy

NA, not applicable.

Adapted and modified from Schug and Bruce (2017).

[1]Difficulty to identify or express one's feelings.

suggestive of neuropathic pain, her treatment with amitriptyline did not help, and the pain was localized, 5% lidocaine plasters were initiated—that is, one plaster every day for 12 consecutive hours by night (U.S. Food and Drug Administration [FDA] and EMA approval for postherpetic neuralgia but recommended for peripheral neuropathic pain by most scientific societies). Other possible drugs would have been gabapentin (300–3600 mg per day, median dosage 1800 mg per day; FDA approval for diabetic painful neuropathy and postherpetic neuralgia; EMA approval for peripheral neuropathic pain) or pregabalin (150–600 mg per day; FDA approval for diabetic painful neuropathy, postherpetic neuralgia, and spinal cord injury pain; EMA approval for neuropathic pain).

This woman now receives 5% lidocaine one plaster per day combined with amitriptyline 75 mg per day, one or two tablets of paracetamol codeine per day, and alprazolam (once a week). Three months after surgery, her postsurgical neuropathic pain is dramatically improved (>70%) and her headache is minimal. You may now consider stopping her topical treatment because she may not develop chronic postsurgical neuropathic pain, probably because of her high-quality pre- and postoperative management.

KEY POINTS TO REMEMBER

- Multiple risk factors for chronic postsurgical pain, including neuropathic pain, have been identified from prospective studies. These include notably preoperative pain, postoperative pain, and opioid use but also many psychological factors, particularly state or trait anxiety, catastrophizing, and depression, as well as lack of cognitive flexibility.
- Patients with these risk factors should be carefully assessed before surgery and monitored after their surgery and managed for their pain as soon as possible to avoid long-term pain chronicization.
- Psychotherapy prior to and after surgery has been found to reduce the risk of chronic postsurgical pain (which is often neuropathic).

Further Reading

Apkarian AV, Baliki MN, Farmer MA. Predicting transition to chronic pain. *Curr Opin Neurol.* 2013;26:360–367.

Attal N, Masselin-Dubois A, Martinez V, et al. Does cognitive functioning predict chronic pain? Results from a prospective surgical cohort. *Brain.* 2014;137:904–917.

Giusti EM, Lacerenza M, Manzoni GM, Castelnuovo G. Psychological and psychosocial predictors of chronic postsurgical pain: A systematic review and meta-analysis. *Pain.* 2021;162(1):10–30.

Masselin-Dubois A, Attal N, Fletcher D, et al. Are psychological predictors of chronic postsurgical pain dependent on the surgical model? A comparison of total knee arthroplasty and breast surgery for cancer. *J Pain.* 2013;14:854–864.

Nadinda PG, van Ryckeghem DML, Peters ML. Can perioperative psychological interventions decrease the risk of post-surgical pain and disability? A systematic review and meta-analysis of randomized controlled trials. *Pain.* 2022;163(7):1254–1273.

Schug SA, Bruce J. Risk stratification for the development of chronic postsurgical pain. *Pain Rep.* 2017;2(6):e627.

35 Management of Patients with Comorbidities

Nadine Attal and Didier Bouhassira

A 42-year-old man complains of severe persisting pain of the lower limb (anterolateral aspect of the thigh) 2 years after surgery for hip arthroplasty. Pain appeared 3 months after surgery and is described as burning, stabbing, shooting, and sensitive to touch. He has a long history of smoking and alcohol consumption, has suffered from several depressive episodes since he was 21 years old, but has never regularly been in psychiatric management. He feels unable to resume his work as property manager. He is getting a difficult divorce because his wife cannot understand him any longer. He expresses anger about his surgeon and a strong feeling of injustice, saying that he was the victim of medical malpractice. He is considering suing his surgeon and, as he says, "I need to be properly reoperated by a good surgeon this time." During the visit, he appears irritated and agitated, and he speaks extremely rapidly, often interrupting you.

What do you do now?

This patient complains of postsurgical pain (pain was not present before surgery) with neuropathic characteristics (it is described as burning, hot, stabbing, shooting, and sensitive to touch), and he has a high score (24) on the PainDETECT questionnaire (neuropathic pain is likely for a cutoff value ≥ 19) (see Chapters 1 and 4). Pain is situated in a neuroanatomical area (the anterolateral aspect of the thigh corresponding to the femoral nerve) and is associated with sensory deficit. The diagnosis of postsurgical neuropathic pain (femoral neuropathy) is probable. In addition to his pain, he reports multiple psychiatric, psychosocial, and somatic comorbidities, which in turn heavily impact his quality of life and work.

First, you have to explain to him that there is no simple relationship between his pain and the nerve lesion, which is a relatively frequent sequelae of surgery and not a sign of surgical malpractice. This may help him understand why reoperation is not justified. Because he has a past history of multiple depressive episodes and is agitated, you may suspect bipolar disorder, but this diagnosis should be confirmed by a psychiatrist. You may tell him that his poor psychological state enhances his disability, reduces the chance of therapeutic success for his postsurgical pain, and that his ongoing divorce and feeling of injustice may also contribute to increase his pain.

After a few weeks, the patient could be referred to a psychiatrist. The diagnosis of bipolar disorder was confirmed, and he was prescribed olanzapine and small dosages of selective serotonin reuptake inhibitor antidepressants. This contributed to reduce his agitation and improve his anxiety, mood, and sleep. After 3 months, the patient is feeling much better but still in pain and walks with difficulty. Now it is possible to orient him to a physical therapist to help him regain some physical activity and reduce his fear of walking. Because he had a well-circumscribed area of pain, capsaicin high-concentration patches were proposed (two patches applied every 3 months, because there was no efficacy of lidocaine plasters) (U.S. Food and Drug Administration approved for diabetic painful neuropathy and postherpetic neuralgia). He soon reports excellent efficacy of this treatment and continues to be followed by a psychiatrist. Of note, other therapeutic options for this patient, theoretically recommended as first line for neuropathic pain, would have been difficult because most of them (tricyclics, gabapentin, or pregabalin) increase weight, and antidepressants such as duloxetine are difficult to use in a bipolar patient without the help of a psychiatrist. Opioids are certainly not an option in his case.

Neuropathic pain strongly impairs quality of life, impacts work productivity, and is often associated with anxiety, depression, disturbed sleep, or catastrophizing. Multiple questionnaires or scales may be helpful to assess these PROs in chronic pain patients (Table 35.1). Conversely, past history

TABLE 35.1 **Common Scales and Questionnaires Recommended for Use in Neuropathic Pain Patients to Assess the Various Dimensions of Pain, Quality of Life, Sleep, Anxiety, Depression, Catastrophizing, and Opioid Abuse**

Scale and Authors	Goal	Scoring and Description
Short Form McGill Pain Questionnaire (SF-MPQ) Melzack 1986	To assess the sensory and affective dimensions of pain	Contains 15 items to assess the sensory dimension of pain (11 items) and the affective dimension of pain (4 items), each rated on categorical scales from 0 to 4.
Brief Pain Inventory (BPI); interference Cleeland and Ryan 1994	To assess interference with pain on several domains	Contains seven numerical rating scales (0–10) to assess the impact of pain on everyday activities, enjoyment with life, sleep, walking ability, relationship with others, mood, normal work; total score 70. The higher the score, the worse the impact of pain.
EuroQol (EQ-5D); VAS Brooks 1996	To briefly assess perceived health status	This is a vertical VAS of 100 mm to assess perceived health from 0 to 100. The higher the score, the better the health status.
Hospital Anxiety and Depression Scale (HADS) Zigmund and Haith 1983	To assess symptoms of anxiety and depression	Items to assess anxiety and depression symptoms; total score 21 for anxiety and 21 for depression. The higher the score, the higher the symptoms. A score ≥8/21 suggests significant disorders.

(*continued*)

TABLE 35.1 **Continued**

Scale and Authors	Goal	Scoring and Description
Pain Catastrophizing Scale (PCS) Sullivan 1995	To assess pain catastrophizing (a negative cognitive–affective response to anticipated or actual pain)	Has been found to assess three dimensions of catastrophizing: amplification, ruminations, and helplessness. Total score 52. The higher the score, the higher the catastrophic thinking.
PROMIS; fatigue, quality of life, depression, anxiety, sleep	PRO To assess fatigue, quality of life, anxiety, depression, sleep	Assesses PROs on distinct categorical scales. Several versions with four, six, or eight items. The higher the score, the higher the impairment.
Opioid risk tool Webster 2005	PRO To measure abuse risk with opioids	Should be administered to patients prior to opioid therapy for pain management. A score ≤3 indicates low risk for opioid abuse, a score of 4–7 indicates moderate risk, and a score ≥8 indicates a high risk for opioid abuse.

PRO, patient-reported outcome; VAS, visual analog scale.
Note: These scales have not been specifically developed for neuropathic pain patients but are validated or recommended for use in this population.
For references see Haanpaa et al. (2011) and https://www.healthmeasures.net/explore-measurem ent systems/promis?AspxAutoDetectCookieSup=

of depression, anxiety, or sleep disorders is common in neuropathic pain. For example, in 182 consecutive patients with peripheral neuropathic pain, it was found that lifetime prevalence of psychiatric comorbidity concerned respectively 39% of the patients with regard to anxiety disorders and 47% with regard to mood disorders, with the two most common psychiatric disorders being generalized anxiety and major depressive episodes. Furthermore depression and anxiety may increase the risk of chronic neuropathic pain after surgery (see Chapter 34). Some patients also report a feeling of injustice, which may also be assessed by questionnaires and is associated with enhanced risk of disability, medication use, and work disability.

KEY POINTS TO REMEMBER

- Neuropathic pain has major impact on quality of life, work productivity, and sleep and may be associated with psychiatric comorbidities. The latter may be caused by pain or may be present before the pain, hence contributing to aggravate the pain.
- Detection of these comorbidities is recommended because this may have significant therapeutic implications: Their medical or psychological management should precede or be concomitant to the management of pain.

Further Reading

Attal N, Lanteri-Minet M, Laurent B, Fermanian J, Bouhassira D. The specific disease burden of neuropathic pain: Results of a French nationwide survey. *Pain*. 2011;152:2836–2843.

Cleeland CS, Ryan KM. Pain assessment: Global use of the Brief Pain Inventory. *Ann Acad Med Singapore*. 1994;23:129–138.

Haanpää M, Attal N, Backonja M, et al. NeuPSIG guidelines on neuropathic pain assessment. *Pain*. 2011;152:14–27.

PROMIS. HealthMeasures. https://www.healthmeasures.net/explore-measurement-systems/promis?AspxAutoDetectCookieSup=

Radat F, Margot-Duclot A, Attal N. Psychiatric co-morbidities in patients with chronic peripheral neuropathic pain: A multicentre cohort study. *Eur J Pain*. 2013;17:1547–1557.

Sullivan MJ, Adams H, Horan S, et al. The role of perceived injustice in the experience of chronic pain and disability: Scale development and validation. *J Occup Rehabil*. 2008;18(3):249–261.

36 Management of Neuropathic Pain: Patient-Reported Outcome Measures

Nadine Attal and Didier Bouhassira

A 68-year-old French man living in Miami has suffered from thoracic postherpetic neuralgia for the past 18 months. He has not been vaccinated against herpes zoster because the primary care physician in France never informed him that a vaccine was available. Now he experiences terrible pain, with burning, frequent paroxysms, and sensitivity to touch, to such an extent that he barely tolerates his T-shirt. His doctor asks him to rate his pain intensity during the past 24 hours on a 0–10 numeric rating scale (NRS). He replies that it is difficult to give a simple rating. After giving it some thought, he reports an average pain score of 9/10. The doctor proposes to treat pain with topical lidocaine. After 1 month, average pain intensity does not seem to have changed much; it is now rated 8/10 on a 0–10 NRS. However, the patient now tolerates wearing a T-shirt.

What do you do now?

This man with postherpetic neuralgia has difficulty providing a single rating for pain and finally rates it as 9/10 on a 0–10 NRS. After treatment with lidocaine plasters during 1 month, the patient reports a similar pain intensity (8/10). The reason why he has difficulty rating pain intensity is probably mainly because he suffers from variable neuropathic symptoms (burning pain, electric shocks, and brush-evoked pain). To assess these pain symptoms more precisely, you may ask this patient to fill out neuropathic pain questionnaires. Those specifically validated for neuropathic pain and commonly used include the Neuropathic Pain Scale (10 symptoms scored on numerical scales [0–10] and one temporal item scored on a categorical scale) and the Neuropathic Pain Symptom Inventory (NPSI); (10 symptoms grouped into five dimensions [burning pain, deep pain, paroxysmal pain, allodynia, and paresthesia/dysesthesia], one item assessing pain duration, and 1 item assessing number of pain paroxysms) (Figure 36.1). In fact, this patient had seen a pain specialist, who asked him to fill out the NPSI before and after his treatment. Results of the NPSI showed that some neuropathic dimensions and symptoms (paroxysmal pain and allodynia) were strongly relieved by lidocaine plasters (Figure 36.1).

What does this imply? Obviously, lidocaine plasters were effective on some of the patient's neuropathic symptoms. Thus, you should not stop lidocaine plasters, contrary to what would be expected from his average pain intensity scores. Instead, you may continue this treatment at similar dosages and add medications for burning pain. Here, because the patient has renal insufficiency and recent myocardial infarction, it is advised to start another topical treatment such as capsaicin high-concentration patch (which has U.S. Food and Drug Administration approval for postherpetic neuralgia)—rather than oral therapy.

This patient is still receiving lidocaine plasters and has started capsaicin high-concentration patches (8%) every 3 months. This treatment contributed to reduce his burning by 50% with acceptable tolerability.

This case shows that neuropathic pain questionnaires may contribute to individualize therapy because they may help assess which neuropathic symptoms can be improved by analgesic treatments. Importantly, most treatments of neuropathic pain have an incomplete effect on pain symptoms. Thus, the use of neuropathic questionnaires in routine may facilitate treatment adaptation. It may also be possible in the future to use

(A) NEUROPATHIC PAIN SYMPTOM INVENTORY

You are suffering from pains due to injury or disease of the nervous system. These pains may be of several types. You may have spontaneous pain, that is pain in the absence of any stimulation, which may be long-lasting or occur as brief attacks. You may also have pain provoked or increased by brushing, pressure, contact with cold or warmth in the painful area. You may feel one or several types of pain. This questionnaire has been developed to help your doctor to better evaluate and treat the various types of pain you feel.

*We wish to know if you feel spontaneous pain, that is pain without any stimulation. For each of the following questions, please select the number that best describes your **average spontaneous pain severity during the past 24 hours.** Select the number 0 if you have not felt such pain. (circle one number only)*

Q1/. Does your pain feel like burning ?

| No burning | 0 | 1 | 2 | 3 | 4 | 5 | 6 | 7 | (8) | 9 | 10 | Worst burning imaginable |

Q2/. Does your pain feel like squeezing ?

| No squeezing | (0) | 1 | 2 | 3 | 4 | 5 | 6 | 7 | 8 | 9 | 10 | Worst squeezing imaginable |

Q3/. Does your pain feel like pressure ?

| No pressure | (0) | 1 | 2 | 3 | 4 | 5 | 6 | 7 | 8 | 9 | 10 | Worst pressure imaginable |

Q4/. **During the past 24 hours,** your spontaneous pain has been present :

Select the response that best describes your case

Permanently	/X/
Between 8 and 12 hours	/ /
Between 4 and 7 hours	/ /
Between 1 and 3 hours	/ /
Less than 1 hour	/ /

*We wish to know if you have brief attacks of pain. For each of the following questions, please select the number that best describes the **average severity of your painful attacks during the past 24 hours.** Select the number 0 if you have not felt such pain. (circle one number only)*

Q5/. Does your pain feel like electric shocks ?

| No electric shocks | 0 | 1 | 2 | 3 | 4 | 5 | 6 | 7 | (8) | 9 | 10 | Worst electric shocks imaginable |

Q6/. Does your pain feel like stabbing ?

| No stabbing | 0 | 1 | 2 | 3 | 4 | 5 | (6) | 7 | 8 | 9 | 10 | Worst stabbing imaginable |

FIGURE 36.1 Results obtained by this patient with postherpetic neuralgia on the Neuropathic Pain Symptom Inventory (NPSI) before and after treatment with 5% lidocaine plasters. The NPSI includes 10 symptoms each rated on 0–10 numerical pain scales (0: no pain, 10: maximal pain imaginable), grouped into five dimensions: burning pain, deep pain (average of squeezing and pressure pain), paroxysmal pain (average of electric shocks and stabbing), evoked pains (average of pain induced by brushing, pressure and cold), and paresthesia/dysesthesia (average of tingling and pins and needles). It also includes two temporal items. Results before treatment (A) were as follows: 8/10 for burning pain, 0/10 for deep pain, 7/10 for paroxysmal pain, 9/10 for evoked pain, and 2/10 for paresthesia. After treatment (B), results became: 7/10 for burning pain, 0 for deep pain, 2/10 for paroxysmal pain, 4/10 for evoked pain, and 2/10 for paresthesia. There was also a consistent decrease in the number of pain paroxysms (item 7). Hence lidocaine plasters alleviated specifically electric shocks and evoked pains.

Q7/. **During the past 24 hours,** how many of these pain attacks have you had ?

Select the response that best describes your case

More than 20	☒
Between 11 and 20	/_/
Between 6 and 10	/_/
Between 1 and 5	/_/
No pain attack	/_/

*We wish to know if you feel pains provoked or increased by brushing, pressure, contact with cold or warmth on the painful area. For each of the following questions, please select the number that best describes the **average severity of your provoked pains during the past 24 hours**. Select the number 0 if you have not felt such pain. (circle one number only)*

Q8/. Is your pain provoked or increased by brushing on the painful area ?

No pain | 0 | 1 | 2 | 3 | 4 | 5 | 6 | 7 | 8 | 9 | (10) | Worst pain imaginable

Q9/. Is your pain provoked or increased by pressure on the painful area ?

No pain | 0 | 1 | 2 | 3 | 4 | 5 | 6 | 7 | (8) | 9 | 10 | Worst pain imaginable

Q10/. Is your pain provoked or increased by **contact** with something cold on the painful area ?

No pain | (0) | 1 | 2 | 3 | 4 | 5 | 6 | 7 | 8 | 9 | 10 | Worst pain imaginable

*We wish to know if you feel abnormal sensations **in the painful area**. For each of the following questions, please select the number that best describes the **average severity of your abnormal sensations during the past 24 hours**. Select the number 0 if your have not felt such sensation. (circle one number only)*

Q11/. Do you feel pins and needles ?

No pins & needles | 0 | 1 | (2) | 3 | 4 | 5 | 6 | 7 | 8 | 9 | 10 | Worst pins & needles imaginable

Q12/. Do you feel tingling ?

No tingling | 0 | 1 | (2) | 3 | 4 | 5 | 6 | 7 | 8 | 9 | 10 | Worst tingling imaginable

---

RESULTS

1 – BURNING (SUPERFICIAL) SPONTANEOUS PAIN	Q1 =	8/10
2 – PRESSING (DEEP) SPONTANEOUS PAIN	(Q2+Q3) /2 =	0/10
3 – PAROXYSMAL PAIN	(Q5+ Q6) /2 =	7/10
4 – EVOKED PAIN	(Q8+Q9+Q10) /3 =	9/10
5 – PARESTHESIA	(Q11+Q12) /2 =	2/10

FIGURE 36.1 Continued

(B) NEUROPATHIC PAIN SYMPTOM INVENTORY

You are suffering from pains due to injury or disease of the nervous system. These pains may be of several types. You may have spontaneous pain, that is pain in the absence of any stimulation, which may be long-lasting or occur as brief attacks. You may also have pain provoked or increased by brushing, pressure, contact with cold or warmth in the painful area. You may feel one or several types of pain. This questionnaire has been developed to help your doctor to better evaluate and treat the various types of pain you feel.

We wish to know if you feel spontaneous pain, that is pain without any stimulation. For each of the following questions, please select the number that best describes your **average spontaneous pain severity during the past 24 hours.** *Select the number 0 if you have not felt such pain. (circle one number only)*

Q1/. Does your pain feel like burning ?

| No burning | 0 | 1 | 2 | 3 | 4 | 5 | 6 | (7) | 8 | 9 | 10 | Worst burning imaginable |

Q2/. Does your pain feel like squeezing ?

| No squeezing | (0) | 1 | 2 | 3 | 4 | 5 | 6 | 7 | 8 | 9 | 10 | Worst squeezing imaginable |

Q3/. Does your pain feel like pressure ?

| No pressure | (0) | 1 | 2 | 3 | 4 | 5 | 6 | 7 | 8 | 9 | 10 | Worst pressure imaginable |

Q4/. **During the past 24 hours,** your spontaneous pain has been present :

Select the response that best describes your case

Permanently	☒
Between 8 and 12 hours	/_/
Between 4 and 7 hours	/_/
Between 1 and 3 hours	/_/
Less than 1 hour	/_/

We wish to know if you have brief attacks of pain. For each of the following questions, please select the number that best describes the **average severity of your painful attacks during the past 24 hours.** *Select the number 0 if you have not felt such pain. (circle one number only)*

Q5/. Does your pain feel like electric shocks ?

| No electric shocks | 0 | 1 | 2 | (3) | 4 | 5 | 6 | 7 | 8 | 9 | 10 | Worst electric shocks imaginable |

Q6/. Does your pain feel like stabbing ?

| No stabbing | 0 | (1) | 2 | 3 | 4 | 5 | 6 | 7 | 8 | 9 | 10 | Worst stabbing imaginable |

FIGURE 36.1 Continued

Q7/. **During the past 24 hours,** how many of these pain attacks have you had ?

Select the response that best describes your case

More than 20	/_/
Between 11 and 20	/_/
Between 6 and 10	/_/
Between 1 and 5	☒
No pain attack	/_/

*We wish to know if you feel pains provoked or increased by brushing, pressure, contact with cold or warmth on the painful area. For each of the following questions, please select the number that best describes the **average severity of your provoked pains during the past 24 hours**. Select the number 0 if you have not felt such pain. (circle one number only)*

Q8/. Is your pain provoked or increased by brushing on the painful area ?

No pain | 0 | 1 | 2 | 3 | (4) | 5 | 6 | 7 | 8 | 9 | 10 | Worst pain imaginable

Q9/. Is your pain provoked or increased by pressure on the painful area ?

No pain | 0 | 1 | 2 | 3 | (4) | 5 | 6 | 7 | 8 | 9 | 10 | Worst pain imaginable

Q10/. Is your pain provoked or increased by **contact** with something cold on the painful area ?

No pain | (0) | 1 | 2 | 3 | 4 | 5 | 6 | 7 | 8 | 9 | 10 | Worst pain imaginable

*We wish to know if you feel abnormal sensations **in the painful area**. For each of the following questions, please select the number that best describes the **average severity of your abnormal sensations during the past 24 hours**. Select the number 0 if your have not felt such sensation. (circle one number only)*

Q11/. Do you feel pins and needles ?

No pins & needles | 0 | 1 | 2 | (3) | 4 | 5 | 6 | 7 | 8 | 9 | 10 | Worst pins & needles imaginable

Q12/. Do you feel tingling ?

No tingling | 0 | (1) | 2 | 3 | 4 | 5 | 6 | 7 | 8 | 9 | 10 | Worst tingling imaginable

---

RESULTS

1 – BURNING (SUPERFICIAL) SPONTANEOUS PAIN .... Q1 =		7/10
2 – PRESSING (DEEP) SPONTANEOUS PAIN .... (Q2+Q3) /2 =		0/10
3 – PAROXYSMAL PAIN ....(Q5+ Q6) /2 =		2/10
4 – EVOKED PAIN .... (Q8+Q9+Q10) /3 =		4/10
5 – PARESTHESIA .... (Q11+Q12) /2 =		2/10

FIGURE 36.1 Continued

these questionnaires to identify individual responder profiles to therapy. These questionnaires are also largely used in multicenter clinical trials of neuropathic pain.

KEY POINTS TO REMEMBER

- Neuropathic symptoms may be assessed by specific neuropathic pain questionnaires.
- These questionnaires may be more sensitive to treatment than global measures of pain intensity and may be used in routine, thus contributing to adapt treatment.
- They may also be relevant to predict outcome of management.

Further Reading

Attal N, Bouhassira D, Baron R. Diagnosis and assessment of neuropathic pain through questionnaires. *Lancet Neurol.* 2018;17:456–466.

Bouhassira D, Branders S, Attal N, et al. Stratification of patients based on the Neuropathic Pain Symptom Inventory: Development and validation of a new algorithm. *Pain.* 2021;162:1038–1046.

Colloca L, Ludman T, Bouhassira D, et al. Neuropathic pain. *Nat Rev Dis Primers.* 2017;3:17002.

37 Management of Neuropathic Pain: Quantitative Sensory Testing

Dilara Kersebaum and Ralf Baron

A 74-year-old female patient with postherpetic neuralgia in the left T1 dermatoma comes to visit you. She has recently been treated with pregabalin (up to 400 mg per day) and then gabapentin (up to 1800 mg per day) with no notable analgesic effect and does not tolerate duloxetine even at low dosages (30 mg per day) because of severe nausea and abdominal pain. Because of pain-associated distress, her primary care physician has added tramadol 50 mg on demand, which she is not looking favorably upon due to possible adverse effects (e.g., addiction and dizziness). She reports no notable medical history. This woman is disturbed by her poor therapeutic results thus far, and she fears another therapeutic failure.

What do you do now?

This woman with postherpetic neuralgia did not benefit from adequate trials of first- or second-line drugs for neuropathic pain. This might be due to multiple reasons, including insufficient dosages and physical or psychological comorbidities. However, one possible reason for therapeutic failure may be that these drugs did not target adequately her symptoms, which involve specific mechanisms. To further select analgesic therapy, you may orient this woman to a specialized center to perform quantitative sensory testing (QST).

QST is a psychophysical method that uses standardized mechanical and thermal stimuli to test the nociceptive and non-nociceptive systems in the periphery and the central nervous system (Figure 37.1; Table 37.1). QST assesses loss of function (hypoesthesia and hypoalgesia) and gain of function

A (= thermotest)

B (= thermode)

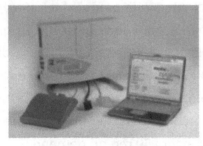
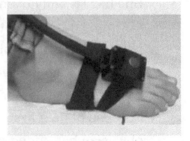

C (= pinprick)

D (= monorilaments)

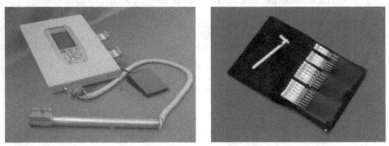

FIGURE 37.1 Common QST equipment. (A) Thermotest using Peltier-type elements to assess detection and pain thresholds to warm and cold stimulation. (B) Photograph of a thermode from Thermotest applied to the subject's dorsum of foot. (C) Pinprick stimulators to assess pain in response to pinprick stimulation. (D) Calibrated monofilaments to asses fine tactile stimuli.

Source: Figure 37.1B courtesy of Ralf Baron (Kiel, Germany).

TABLE 37.1 Normative Values, Advantages, and Limitations of QST

Normative values	Age- and sex-matched database for absolute and relative QST reference data is available for healthy human subjects (German Network on Neuropathic Pain).
Advantages	Detects sensory deficits and thermal deficits, which may be an initial sign of small fiber neuropathy. Monitors the outcome of sensory neuropathies or sensory deficits. Assesses pain modulation (using a method called conditioned pain modulation). Assesses the sensory profile of patients (variable combinations of sensory deficits and evoked pains) allowing to subgroup patients based on potential mechanisms and adapt the treatment. Recommended by the European Medicines Agency for exploratory trials on neuropathic pain.
Limitations	Expensive. Requires extensive training. Very lengthy if using the full German protocol (bedside testing protocols may now overcome this issue). Difficult to establish at individual level whether results are pathological or not. QST is not a stand-alone test, and results should be analyzed in the context of other investigations. Assesses evoked pain (allodynia, hyperalgesia) but not spontaneous pain (e.g., burning), which may be best assessed with questionnaires (it is possible to combine QST and questionnaires to stratify patients in clinical trials and aim for a personalized approach to neuropathic pain).

Adapted and modified from Backonja et al. (2013).

(allodynia and hyperalgesia) of all the different afferent fiber classes. Its main advantages over standard clinical examination is that the stimulus is controlled, which allows quantification of the severity of hypoesthesia or conversely allodynia and hyperalgesia (and not simply to check whether the deficit or evoked pain is present or absent).

Here, results showed that this woman has very limited thermal and mechanical deficit and instead has severe cold allodynia and allodynia to brush (dynamic mechanical allodynia). Although not possible to directly confirm,

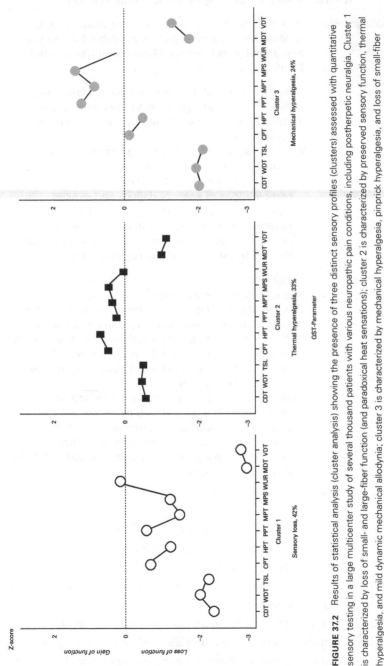

FIGURE 37.2 Results of statistical analysis (cluster analysis) showing the presence of three distinct sensory profiles (clusters) assessed with quantitative sensory testing in a large multicenter study of several thousand patients with various neuropathic pain conditions, including postherpetic neuralgia. Cluster 1 is characterized by loss of small- and large-fiber function (and paradoxical heat sensations); cluster 2 is characterized by preserved sensory function, thermal hyperalgesia, and mild dynamic mechanical allodynia; cluster 3 is characterized by mechanical hyperalgesia, pinprick hyperalgesia, and loss of small-fiber function. It is presumable that each cluster reflects specific mechanisms and may respond to specific therapies.

Reproduced with permission from Baron et al. (2017).

this suggests that the mechanisms involved in her pain mainly result from peripheral mechanisms (e.g., pathological spontaneous discharges in nociceptive fibers and lowered activation threshold for thermal/mechanical stimuli) (Figure 37.2).

In this case, rather than gabapentin, pregabalin, or duloxetine, which act on central targets, it may be relevant to propose drugs acting mainly on peripheral mechanisms. Among recommended drugs for postherpetic neuralgia, topical lidocaine, a local sodium channel blocker acting specifically on peripheral mechanisms, is the most rationale option and has approval for use in postherpetic neuralgia. Lidocaine plasters have very few side effects—except for a potential risk of cutaneous allergy—and very few contraindications. They should not be proposed for acute herpes zoster because they need to be applied on healthy skin to avoid systemic absorption. It is also advisable to avoid them in patients receiving antiarrhythmic agents such as mexiletine. Generally, one to three plasters have to be applied to the painful area for 12 hours per day.

This woman was treated with 5% lidocaine plasters (two plasters per day during 12 hours per day during daytime). She had no side effects and reported excellent efficacy of lidocaine plasters on her evoked pain, which decreased by 70%. One year later, the efficacy of topical lidocaine decreased concomitantly to severe depression because of major family issues. She then was referred to a psychiatrist, who added fluoxetine 20 mg per day to her therapeutic regimen. As her depression improved, her pain intensity also decreased, and she continues to be treated with fluoxetine and lidocaine plasters.

This case demonstrates the potential advantages of QST from a therapeutic standpoint. However, it also highlights that therapeutic success in neuropathic pain is not just dependent on sensory profile. Obviously, any chronic pain, including postherpetic neuralgia, may be influenced by psychological, social, and genetic factors that may hamper therapeutic efficacy.

KEY POINTS TO REMEMBER

- QST is a psychophysical method allowing the quantification of hypoesthesia, allodynia, and hyperalgesia, and it may be best combined with specific questionnaires to assess symptoms of spontaneous pain.

- Studies using QST have shown that within a single neuropathic pain etiology, signs and symptoms may be related to distinct mechanisms, which may be best targeted by distinct therapeutic agents.
- These data suggest that patient stratification based on QST and questionnaires represents an important step toward the identification of treatment responders in clinical practice and in clinical trials.

Further Reading

Backonja MM, Attal N, Baron R, et al. Value of quantitative sensory testing in neurological and pain disorders: NeuPSIG consensus. *Pain*. 2013;154:1807–1819.

Bannister K, Sachau J, Baron R, Dickenson AH. Neuropathic pain: Mechanism-based therapeutics. *Annu Rev Pharmacol Toxicol*. 2020;60:257–274.

Baron R, Binder A, Wasner G. Neuropathic pain: Diagnosis, pathophysiological mechanisms, and treatment. *Lancet Neurol*. 2010;9(8):807–819.

Baron R, Maier C, Attal N, et al. Peripheral neuropathic pain: A mechanism-related organizing principle based on sensory profiles. *Pain*. 2017;158:261–272.

Baron R, Tölle TR, Gockel U, Brosz M, Freynhagen R. A cross-sectional cohort survey in 2100 patients with painful diabetic neuropathy and postherpetic neuralgia: Differences in demographic data and sensory symptoms. *Pain*. 2009;146:34–40.

Demant DT, Lund K, Vollert J, et al. The effect of oxcarbazepine in peripheral neuropathic pain depends on pain phenotype: A randomised, double-blind, placebo-controlled phenotype-stratified study. *Pain*. 2014;155:2263–2273.

Gierthmühlen J, Schneider U, Seemann M, et al. Can self-reported pain characteristics and bedside test be used for the assessment of pain mechanisms? An analysis of results of neuropathic pain questionnaires and quantitative sensory testing. *Pain*. 2019;160:2093–2104.

Koulouris AE, Edwards RR, Dorado K, et al. Reliability and validity of the Boston Bedside Quantitative Sensory Testing Battery for neuropathic pain. *Pain Med*. 2020;21:2336–2347.

Reimer M, Sachau J, Forstenpointner J, Baron R. Bedside testing for precision pain medicine. *Curr Opin Support Palliat Care*. 2021;15:116–124.

Rolke R, Baron R, Maier C, et al. Quantitative sensory testing in the German Research Network on Neuropathic Pain (DFNS): Standardized protocol and reference values. *Pain*. 2006;123:231–243.

38 Complementary Investigations

Andrea Truini and Eleonora Galosi

A 45-year-old otherwise healthy woman complains of intense leg pain, which developed gradually during the past 6 months. She describes ongoing burning pain involving both soles of the feet ("as if my feet were immersed in boiling water"). Pain is continuous, but it tends to be more severe at night, affecting sleep, associated with tingling, dizziness, and lightheadedness when standing up from a lying position. The neurological examination shows normal coordination and motor function; deep tendon reflexes are normal, although ankle reflexes are mildly diminished. Sensory examination shows no abnormalities in tactile, vibration sensitivity or proprioception. Electromyography with nerve conduction study is normal. Several doctors told her that her pain was "in her head" and that she had fibromyalgia or somatoform disorders (one of them realized that she suffered from moral harassment at work: "This is the cause of your pain!" he said). She was oriented to a psychiatrist, who stated that she does not have a psychiatric condition.

What do you do now?

This woman does not seem to have a psychiatric condition. Based on quality of pain, pain distribution, and sensory examination, aided by complementary investigations, you will probably be able to make a better diagnosis:

1. Her chronic pain is mainly described as burning and associated with tingling. The score obtained with the DN4 interview (seven items) was 3 out of 7 (burning 1, cold 1, tingling 1) (see Chapter 1). This strongly suggests neuropathic pain.
2. Her pain is not widespread over the body as in fibromyalgia but, rather, is symmetric and bilateral, limited to both soles of the feet from the tip of the toes to the area immediately anterior to the heels. This distribution is compatible with that of a sensory polyneuropathy.
3. Her neurological examination seems normal but was incomplete. You should conduct a further sensory examination, using a pinprick and/or cold tube. This test found decreased pinprick and cold sensation limited to the soles. This indicates thermoalgesic deficits. Motor, tendon reflexes, proprioceptive, and tactile deficits indicate an impairment of large myelinated fibers (Aβ fibers mediate light touch, vibration sense, and proprioception; Aα neurons innervate skeletal muscles), whereas thermoalgesic deficits (deficits in cold and warm sensation, decreased or absent cold and heat pain, and reduced pinprick sensation) indicate impairment of small fibers (small myelinated Aδ and unmyelinated C fibers).

Thus, this woman's clinical presentation (bilateral and symmetric neuropathic pain distribution at the feet and thermoalgesic deficit in the same area) is compatible with painful distal symmetric neuropathy with selective involvement of small fibers, a condition referred to as small fiber neuropathy (see Chapter 14). She also complains of dizziness and lightheadedness when standing up. This suggests orthostatic intolerance. You should assess her blood pressure at a lying or sitting position and then a standing position. In this woman, systolic blood pressure dropped 25 mmHg within 3 minutes of standing, with respect to the basal blood pressure from the sitting position. This confirmed orthostatic hypotension, suggesting an impairment of autonomic nerve fibers, which are also small fibers (the autonomic nervous system regulates a number of bodily functions, including heart rate, digestion, respiratory rate, pupillary response, urination, and sexual arousal).

In this woman, EMG was normal. The nerve conduction study (NCS) is the reference standard technique for peripheral neuropathies such as those related to diabetes. However, nerve conduction tests investigate only large myelinated Aβ fibers (see above) and not small fibers. Thus, they may be normal, which is also in favor of small fiber neuropathy. To confirm small fiber sensory neuropathy, you should refer her to a specialized neurological or neurophysiological unit. The most widely agreed-upon methods for investigating small fiber damage are laser evoked potentials and skin biopsy (the method of reference) (Figure 38.1, Table 38.1). Additional tests may include quantitative sensory testing (see Chapter 37) to quantify thermal deficits (but there are false-positive and false-negative results) and corneal confocal microscopy, an ophthalmologic examination of corneal nerve fibers, which has mainly been validated for diabetic neuropathy.

In this woman, laser evoked potential recordings showed abnormally reduced amplitude at the foot, and skin punch biopsy disclosed a reduction in intraepidermal nerve fiber density at the distal calf (below the fifth centile relative to age- and gender-matched controls). These investigations, together with normal NCS, confirmed small fiber neuropathy. You may now search for causes of small fiber neuropathy with dysautonomia (Table 38.1). Recommended biological testings include fasting glycemia, complete blood count, sedimentation level, liver enzymes, immunologic testing (nuclear and DNA antibodies), and, depending on the context, HIV serology. In this woman, this first round of testing was normal. Then you should ask for second-line investigations in specialized centers, including genetic testing for rare pathogenetic voltage-gated sodium channels and transthyretin gene mutations (see Chapter 26).

Before waiting for the results, we advise you treat her pain. Because pain was restricted to the soles, this woman was initially treated by lidocaine plasters (one plaster per foot for 12 consecutive hours a day; FDA and EMA approval for postherpetic neuralgia). Because her pain was only moderately relieved, oral duloxetine (FDA and EMA approved for diabetic painful neuropathy) was initiated at 30 mg daily during meal then increased after 1 week to 60 mg per day, which further improved her neuropathic pain (by 50%). Eventually, genetic testing showed a pathogenetic mutation of the

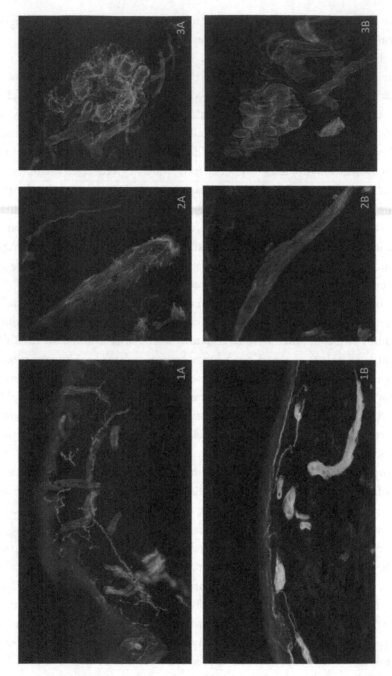

FIGURE 38.1 Skin biopsy findings in a healthy subject (A) and in the patient with small-fiber neuropathy hereditary transthyretin amyloidosis (B). PGP9.5 immunostaining for nerve fibers is marked in red; collagen IV immunostaining is marked in green. The skin biopsy shows severe reduction of intraepidermal nerve fibers density (1B), as well as piloerector muscle (2B) and sweat gland (3B) innervation.

TABLE 38.1 Clinical Description, Main Causes of Small Fiber Neuropathies, and Usually Recommended Complementary Investigations for Assessing Small Fiber Function or Anatomy

Clinical description	Symptoms: neuropathic pain, usually described as burning or prickling Examination: hypoesthesia to pinprick, cold or warm; conversely, evoked pain (allodynia, hyperalgesia) in a distal "stock and glove " distribution Autonomic nervous system dysfunction is common (orthostatic hypotension, gastrointestinal or sexual dysfunction).
Main causes	Diabetes Alcohol Dysimmune conditions: Sjögren syndrome, systemic lupus erythematosus, sarcoidosis Infections: HIV, hepatitis Vitamin deficiency (B_{12}, folate, B_1) Hypothyroidism Genetic: channelopathies; hereditary transthyretin amyloidosis Often no cause is found: these conditions are labeled idiopathic small fiber neuropathies.
Laser evoked potentials	Laser-generated radiant heat pulses selectively excite Aδ and C nociceptors in the superficial skin layers and evoke scalp potentials generated by pain-related brain areas (somatosensory area, insular cortex, and anterior cingulate cortex).
Skin punch biopsy	Consists of a 3-mm-diameter punch, with no need for sutures at a distal site on the leg. Quantifies intraepidermal nerve fiber density (mainly unmyelinated C-fiber terminals and a few Aδ fibers, which lose their myelin sheath and reach the epidermis as unmyelinated free nerve endings). Antibodies against protein gene product 9.5 (PGP 9.5), a pan-axonal marker, allow staining and quantification of intraepidermal nerve fiber density in the collected skin sample. Side effects mainly consist of transient pain and sometimes bleeding and skin discoloration.

transthyretin gene (Val30Met) in favor of hereditary amyloidosis. She received a specific treatment by tafamidis. After 1 year, she was able to discontinue all her analgesic drug treatments and is now pain-free.

KEY POINTS TO REMEMBER

- Small fiber neuropathy is characterized by selective impairment of small thermonociceptive and autonomic fibers, often leading to distally distributed neuropathic pain and thermal pain sensory abnormalities, as well as autonomic dysfunction.
- Specific diagnostic testing for assessing small fibers, such as laser evoked potential recording and skin biopsy, as well as autonomic function testing, is required for diagnosis because nerve conduction study shows no abnormalities in patients with small fiber neuropathy.
- A comprehensive laboratory assessment should be carried out in patients with small fiber neuropathy, aiming at identifying metabolic, autoimmune, inflammatory, and infectious diseases. Genetic testing for rare pathogenetic voltage-gated sodium channels and transthyretin gene mutations should be performed in idiopathic cases.

Further Reading

Colloca L, Ludman T, Bouhassira D, et al. Neuropathic pain. *Nat Rev Dis Primers*. 2017;3:17002.

Devigili G, Rinaldo S, Lombardi R, et al. Diagnostic criteria for small fibre neuropathy in clinical practice and research. *Brain*. 2019;142(12):3728–3736.

Di Stefano G, La Cesa S, Leone C, et al. Diagnostic accuracy of laser-evoked potentials in diabetic neuropathy. *Pain*. 2017;158(6):1100–1107.

Terkelsen AJ, Karlsson P, Lauria G, Freeman R, Finnerup NB, Jensen TS. The diagnostic challenge of small fibre neuropathy: Clinical presentations, evaluations, and causes. *Lancet Neurol*. 2017;16(11):934–944.

Themistocleous AC, Ramirez JD, Serra J, Bennett DL. The clinical approach to small fibre neuropathy and painful channelopathy. *Pract Neurol*. 2014;14(6):368–379.

39 The Case of Cannabinoids

Nadine Attal and Didier Bouhassira

A 47-year-old woman with relapsing–remitting multiple sclerosis suffers from neuropathic pain involving the right hemibody and left face. Pain is reported to be paroxysmal with severe electric shocks up to 20 times a day. Paroxysms are unpredictable, have no trigger, and are often associated with painful tonic spasms of the right leg (brief, painful unilateral muscle contractions lasting 30 seconds to 3 minutes). Pain has not responded to pregabalin, gabapentin, duloxetine, nortriptyline, tramadol, and sustained-release morphine. She tells you that the only treatment which she finds beneficial for her paroxysmal pain is smoking cannabis (she smokes up to 10 cigarettes per day). She has no signs of craving (no strong desire for the drug other than for pain relief) but is afraid of being dependent. She is not depressed. She also now suffers from chronic bronchopathy due to long-standing smoking use.

What do you do now?

This woman has central neuropathic pain related to multiple sclerosis, which is refractory to first-, second-, and third-line antineuropathic medications. She smokes cannabis with good efficacy on her pain paroxysms and tonic spasms. She does not have signs of craving. This is a good indication to start oral or sublingual cannabinoids, after psychiatrist advice and close monitoring, which may also help her reduce smoked cannabis.

Cannabis-based medicines are pharmaceutical products containing tetrahydrocannabinol (THC), cannabidiol (CBD), or a combination of both (Table 39.1). To date, main cannabinoids for pain (although not approved for this indication) are oral THC (dronabinol), U.S. Food and Drug Administration (FDA) approved for anorexia associated with weight loss in AIDS patients; oral nabilone (or Cesamet; synthetically derived from THC), FDA approved for nausea associated with cancer chemotherapy; and nabiximols (Sativex), a THC:CBD oromucosal spray (2.7 mg THC/2.5 mg CBD), approved for spasticity associated with multiple sclerosis (in Canada and the United Kingdom) but not FDA approved. CBD is nearly devoid of psychoactive risks and is available in many countries and also many U.S. states under different forms (oils and sometimes vaporization). It does not have the status of a medicinal drug. Unfortunately, it has little efficacy for pain and is mainly helpful for mild anxiety or well-being.

This woman started on oral THC 2.5 mg per day and titrated up to 20 mg TID by steps of 2.5 mg every 3 days, while progressively reducing smoked cannabis. After a few weeks, the treatment alleviated her pain paroxysms by 70% and she was able to stop smoking cannabis. She did not develop dependency to oral THC. She remains closely monitored by her physician. Another option, depending on availability, would have been sublingual nabiximols (2.7 mg THC and 2.5 mg CBD per spray) titrated progressively up to 10 sprays per day, corresponding to 27 mg of THC and 25 mg CBD per day. You should advise her of potential adverse effects of cannabinoids, including dizziness, dry mouth, disorientation, nausea, euphoria, confusion, and somnolence. A major concern is the potential risk of psychosis and of cannabis dependency, particularly in adolescents. Contraindications include recent stroke, ongoing cardiopathy, severe renal or hepatic insufficiency, and psychosis.

TABLE 39.1 **Terminology and Definitions of Cannabinoids**[a]

Term and Examples	Definition
Herbal cannabis Cannabis sativa, hashish	Whole plant or parts of the plant (flowers, buds, resin, leaves, etc.); contains terpenes, flavonoids, and other compounds, which are probably pharmacologically active
Medical or medicinal cannabis or marijuana Tilray/Aurora 25 THC/25 CBD	Cannabis plants, plant material, or full plant extracts used for medical purposes
Cannabinoids THC, CBD, nabilone	Biologically active constituents of cannabis or synthetic compounds with affinity for cannabinoid receptors
Cannabis-based (or cannabis-derived) medicines Nabiximols (Sativex), dronabinol (Marinol), Epidiolex	Medicinal cannabis extracts or products with regulatory approval for therapeutic purposes with standardized THC and/or CBD content
Phytocannabinoids THC, CBD	Cannabinoids found in cannabis plants or purified/extracted from plant materials
Endocannabinoids Anandamide	Endogenous ligands with affinity for cannabinoid receptors
Cannabinoid receptor antagonists Ribonabant	Block cannabinoid receptors via action of endogenous ligands
Modulators that increase or enhance endocannabinoid system activity FAAH inhibitors	Other drugs (under development) acting on endocannabinoid systems, such as cannabinoid receptor agonists, or inhibitors of cannabinoid catabolism (FAAH inhibitors)

[a]The analgesic efficacy of cannabinoids is mainly driven by THC, the psychoactive compound of cannabis, through agonist activity at cannabinoid type 1 (CB1) and type 2 (CB2) receptors. CB1 receptors are widely distributed in the central nervous system, including the pain descending pathway, dorsal horn of the spinal cord, and dorsal root ganglion, whereas CB2 receptors are mainly found in peripheral nerve endings and in the immune system. Cannabinoids also include endocannabinoid modulators; the endocannabinoid system also represents a therapeutic target for chronic pain.

CBD, cannabidiol; FAAH, fatty acid amide hydrolase; THC, Δ^9-tetrahydrocannabinol.

Adapted from Soliman et al. (2021).

Cannabinoids are widely used for neuropathic pain in several countries worldwide, with large-scale published registries showing that they may be safe and effective. The efficacy of cannabinoids is well documented for painful spasticity in multiple sclerosis. In neuropathic pain, oromucosal cannabinoids (nabiximols, 7 mg THC and 25 mg CBD per milliliter) and oral dronabinol (10–40 mg per day) have been most commonly assessed, but results are variable (among 11 placebo controlled trials of cannabinoids administered for >3 weeks, only 3 are positive). Best evidence for efficacy of cannabinoids stems from short-term studies of smoked cannabis in HIV neuropathy (generally 1 week). However, based on open-label studies, cannabinoids seem particularly effective for pain paroxysms (electric shocks and stabbing pain).

KEY POINTS TO REMEMBER

- Cannabinoids have been more studied in neuropathic pain than in other types of chronic pain. The main cannabinoids investigated include smoked cannabis, oral THC, and nabiximols (oromucosal THC:CBD).
- Although smoked cannabis appears to be effective on a short-term basis, results of randomized controlled trials of other cannabinoids administered for more than 3 weeks are inconclusive. However, large-scale registries suggest their efficacy and safety in many patients with neuropathic pain.
- Based on open-label studies, cannabinoids seem to be more effective on neuropathic pain paroxysms.

Further Reading

Attal N, Bouhassira D. Advances in the treatment of neuropathic pain. *Curr Opin Neurol.* 2021;34(5):631–637.

Finnerup NB, Attal N, Haroutounian S, et al. Pharmacotherapy for neuropathic pain in adults: A systematic review and meta-analysis. *Lancet Neurol.* 2015;14(2):162–173.

Häuser W, Petzke F, Fitzcharles MA. Efficacy, tolerability and safety of cannabis-based medicines for chronic pain management—An overview of systematic reviews. *Eur J Pain.* 2018;22(3):455–470.

Moisset X, Bouhassira D, Avez Couturier J, et al. Pharmacological and non-pharmacological treatments for neuropathic pain: Systematic review and French recommendations. *Rev Neurol*. 2020;176(5):325–352.

Soliman N, Haroutounian S, Hohmann AG, et al. Systematic review and meta-analysis of cannabinoids, cannabis-based medicines, and endocannabinoid system modulators tested for antinociceptive effects in animal models of injury-related or pathological persistent pain. *Pain*. 2021;162(Suppl 1):S26–S44.

40 Nerve Blocks and Drug Infusions

Benjamin Portal, Ravneet Bhullar, and Charles Argoff

A 30-year-old woman without significant past medical history presents with persistent right ankle pain following a sprain without fracture 13 months ago. The orthopedic surgeon believes that her sprain has healed and has no explanation for the pain. Examination reveals tactile and cold thermal allodynia over the right ankle and foot; diminished pinprick and vibratory sensation on the right distal, medial, and lateral leg; shiny, cool skin with bluish discoloration; limited dorsiflexion, plantar flexion, and foot inversion and eversion; 4/5 strength of dorsiflexion, plantar flexion, and inversion and eversion; and thinning of the nails of the right foot. Pain persists despite appropriate medical management including gabapentin and corticosteroids for a short period. Psychotherapy has helped her better cope with pain but did not change pain intensity. Physiotherapy was advised but extremely difficult to implement because of pain generated by each exercise and the patient felt discouraged.

What do you do now?

This patient fulfills clinical criteria for complex regional pain syndrome (CRPS) (Chapter 9). Because CRPS may be due in part to autonomic dysregulation with an exaggerated response to catecholamines, sympathetic nerve blocks have largely been utilized for this condition. However, although routinely used and despite multiple case reports, their long-term efficacy has not been confirmed. This woman received repeated regional somatic anesthetic blocks to help her participate in physical therapy. Then these blocks were stopped and rehabilitation was continued under oral opioid therapy (10 mg oral morphine 1 hour before each physical therapy session). She was progressively able to recover function and her pain improved, although her range of motion remains partially limited.

Regional somatic nerve blocks using local anesthetics (lidocaine, bupivacaine, and ropivacaine, which act as sodium channel blockers) (Table 40.1) have been proposed for patients with CRPS or focal painful nerve injuries, such as postsurgical nerve lesions (e.g., ilioinguinal nerve lesions after hernia repair and post-mastectomy or post-thoracotomy pain syndromes). Occipital nerve blocks have also been found beneficial for occipital neuralgia (Chapter 43). With the exception of occipital neuralgia, the sustained efficacy of somatic nerve blocks is not demonstrated in neuropathic pain or CRPS, which makes it difficult to recommend them as stand-alone treatments. These blocks may mainly be useful for diagnostic purposes (to show the contribution of a specific nerve in neuropathic pain) or to facilitate rehabilitation in the case of CRPS. Clinicians should be advised of their potential systemic effects, which are mainly neurological or cardiac.

TABLE 40.1 **Main Local Anesthetics Used for Somatic Nerve Blocks**

Anesthetic	Relative Local Anaesthetic Potency	Onset of Action (Minutes)	Duration of Action (Hours)	Toxicity
Lidocaine	1	5–10	1.5	Neurological
Bupivacaine	4	10–30	6–12	Mainly cardiac
Ropivacaine	4	10–20	6–14	Cardiac

Among intravenous (IV) analgesic infusions, those of ketamine (0.15–2 mg/kg during 90 minutes), an *N*-nitrosodimethylamine (NDMA) antagonist (NMDA receptors are involved in central sensitization), and the sodium channel blocker lidocaine (3–7.5 mg/kg IV during 90 minutes) have been explored in refractory neuropathic pain, with several studies reporting their short-term efficacy for up to 2 weeks after the infusion. However, placebo-controlled studies assessing their longer term efficacy (3 or 5 weeks) are generally negative. Thus, these infusions need to be repeated over time for sustained efficacy, which makes them impossible to use in most cases in routine care (except in rare patients reporting a long duration of effects or to relieve pain exacerbations). Side effects of ketamine include dissociation, somnolence, and dizziness (which can be attenuated by benzodiazepine premedication); common side effects of lidocaine include drowsiness, dizziness, and fatigue, but there may be potential cardiac and neurological toxicity. Hence, administration of these drugs requires close cardiovascular monitoring in specialized centers, preferably in post-anesthesia care units. None of these treatments are approved for use in chronic pain.

KEY POINTS TO REMEMBER

- Sympathetic nerve blocks are routinely used for CRPS, but evidence based on adequate studies is lacking regarding their efficacy.
- Regional analgesic blockade with local anesthetics can be used mainly to facilitate physical therapy or for diagnostic purposes in CRPS or peripheral neuropathic pain patients.
- Intravenous infusions of ketamine or lidocaine have been found beneficial in neuropathic pain mainly for a short period (<3 weeks after the infusion). They may be recommended after medical concertation for a few patients with refractory pain to relieve severe pain exacerbations.

Further Reading

Birklein F, Neill D, Schlereth T. Complex regional pain syndrome: An optimistic perspective. *Neurology*. 2015;84(1):89–96.

Harden RN, Oaklander AL, Burton AW, et al.; Reflex Sympathetic Dystrophy
Syndrome Association. Complex regional pain syndrome: Practical diagnostic
and treatment guidelines, 4th edition. *Pain Med.* 2013;14(2):180–229.

Kissoon NR, O'Brien TG, Bendel MA, et al. Comparative Effectiveness of Landmark-
guided Greater Occipital Nerve (GON) Block at the Superior Nuchal Line Versus
Ultrasound-guided GON Block at the Level of C2: A Randomized Clinical Trial
(RCT). *Clin J Pain.* 2022;38(4):271–278.

O'Connell NE, Wand BM, Gibson W, Carr DB, Birklein F, Stanton TR. Local anaesthetic
sympathetic blockade for complex regional pain syndrome. *Cochrane Database
Syst Rev.* 2016;7(7):CD004598.

Pickering G, Pereira B, Morel V, et al. Ketamine and magnesium for refractory
neuropathic pain: A randomized, double-blind, crossover trial. *Anesthesiology.*
2020;133(1):154–164.

Urits I, Shen AH, Jones MR, Viswanath O, Kaye AD. Complex regional pain
syndrome, current concepts and treatment options. *Curr Pain Headache Rep.*
2018;22(2):10.

Veizi IE, Chelimsky TC, Janata JW. Chronic regional pain syndrome: What
specialized rehabilitation services do patients require? *Curr Pain Headache Rep.*
2012;16:139–146.

Xu J, Herndon C, Anderson S, et al. Intravenous ketamine infusion for complex
regional pain syndrome: Survey, consensus, and a reference protocol. *Pain Med.*
2019;20(2):323–334.

41 Noninvasive Brain Stimulation

Nadine Attal and Didier Bouhassira

A 73-year-old woman suffers from severe facial pain after surgery for brainstem meningioma. Pain covers the V2 and V3 right territory and is reported to be continuous, described as burning and shooting, and is associated with severe numbness, tingling, and pins and needles. Average pain intensity is 7/10. There are no electric shocks. Examination discloses anesthesia of the painful area. A diagnosis of symptomatic trigeminal neuralgia secondary to her brainstem lesion is posed. A number of drug treatments have been attempted, including gabapentin, pregabalin, carbamazepine, duloxetine, amitriptylin, and oxycodone, but they were generally poorly tolerated. Lidocaine plasters and transcutaneous electrical nerve stimulation are totally ineffective (she does not feel the tingling induced by electrodes). Thermocoagulation (of the Gasser ganglion) is not an option because her pain is present in an area of severe sensory deficit.

What do you do now?

This woman suffers from symptomatic trigeminal neuralgia with continuous facial pain, no pain paroxysms, and anesthesia of the painful area. This clinical picture should not be confused with idiopathic or classical trigeminal neuralgia, in which the standard neurological examination is normal (Chapter 19). She has not responded to first- or second-line drugs for neuropathic pain. She may be referred for noninvasive central brain stimulation in specialized centers. These techniques encompass repeated high-frequency (≥10 Hz) repetitive transcranial magnetic stimulation (rTMS) (Figure 41.1A) and transcranial direct current stimulation (tDCS).

After ensuring for the lack of contraindication, this woman was referred for rTMS of the motor cortex in a specialized hospital center. The following protocol was simplified from published studies (and efficacy was suggested in routine in more than 400 patients treated in a French university hospital center). Parameters of stimulation are 1,500–3,000 pulses per session, frequency 10 Hz, 80% of the motor threshold, and total duration 20 minutes per session. Total number of sessions is 10 over a 6-month period. This includes 3 daily sessions for 3 consecutive days, 1 rTMS session per week during the next 3 weeks, and then 5 monthly sessions. The analgesic benefit of the first 5 rTMS sessions is assessed at 1 month. If there is no efficacy (<30% pain relief or no improvement of quality of life or clinical global impression of change), treatment is stopped. This woman underwent 5 repeated rTMS sessions during 1 month. After these 5 rTMS sessions, she reported 30% benefit on pain and felt "much improved." It was decided to continue the treatment. She finally received 6 months of rTMS sessions (a total of 10 sessions since the beginning of therapy) with excellent safety and efficacy on her pain (70%), and she continues to receive 1 rTMS session every 3 months with ongoing efficacy. Long-term efficacy of infrequent rTMS sessions (every 3–6 months) has sometimes been reported in routine use or anecdotal reports, but this needs to be confirmed by well-designed studies.

Efficacy of repeated sessions of rTMS of the left motor cortex (the motor cortex being considered as the most effective target to date in analgesia) has been reported in placebo-controlled randomized controlled studies in neuropathic pain, including a recent French multicenter study showing maintenance of efficacy for 6 months. The site of stimulation is generally contralateral to the area of pain or left in bilateral pain. Recent studies used robotic-assisted neuronavigation and double-face coil (with an active and

(a)

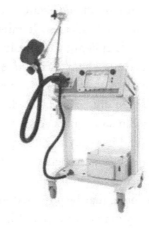

(b)

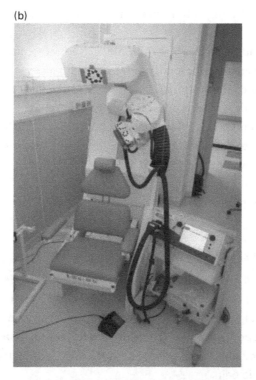

FIGURE 41.1 Photographs of the rTMS device (A) and of a robot used to maintain the coil (Axilum Robotics) (B).

a placebo face) to ensure blinding (Figure 41.1B). rTMS is generally well tolerated except for minor headaches. It rarely induces seizures. Relative contraindications include epilepsy, and absolute contraindications are deep brain electrodes and cochlear implants. There are several published rTMS protocols in analgesia, but in all cases it is necessary to repeat the sessions (generally four or five) to obtain an analgesic effect, and effects may last 1 month or more between subsequent sessions. Efficacy is observed at high frequency (≥ 10 Hz) and intensity (>500 pulses per session) (studies using low frequency or intensity are generally negative). Mechanisms probably involve central modulatory controls and/or brain neuroplasticity changes. rTMS of the motor cortex may be proposed for patients with chronic neuropathic pain refractory to first- and second-line medications. It is currently approved in Europe (European Medicines Agency) and the United States (U.S. Food and Drug Administration) for major depression, but not in analgesia.

tDCS is another technique of noninvasive brain stimulation. It uses a battery-powered device that transfers low-intensity electrical current to the surface of the scalp. It is much less costly than rTMS. tDCS of the motor cortex has been proposed for refractory neuropathic pain and induces only minor side effects (mainly headache and pain at the stimulation site), with cumulative effects over multiple sessions, as is the case for rTMS. However, the level of evidence for efficacy is weaker than for rTMS. Novel rTMS techniques such as "deep rTMS" or theta burst rTMS are also promising.

KEY POINTS TO REMEMBER

- rTMS of the motor cortex has been found effective for peripheral and central refractory neuropathic pain in well-designed placebo-controlled, randomized controlled trials.
- Safety is good, with the main side effect being headache.
- The efficacy of tDCS of the motor cortex is less established for neuropathic pain.
- Newer targets and parameters of stimulation are currently being investigated.

Further Reading

Attal N, Ayache SS, Ciampi De Andrade D, et al. Repetitive transcranial magnetic stimulation and transcranial direct-current stimulation in neuropathic pain due to radiculopathy: A randomized sham-controlled comparative study. *Pain.* 2016;157(6):1224–1231.

Attal N, Poindessous-Jazat F, De Chauvigny E, et al. Repetitive transcranial magnetic stimulation for neuropathic pain: A randomized multicentre sham-controlled trial. *Brain.* 2021;144(11):3328–3339.

Knotkova H, Hamani C, Sivanesan E, Le Beuffe MFE, Moon JY, Cohen SP, Huntoon MA. Neuromodulation for chronic pain. *Lancet.* 2021;397(10289):2111–2124.

Lefaucheur JP, Aleman A, Baeken C, et al. Evidence-based guidelines on the therapeutic use of repetitive transcranial magnetic stimulation (rTMS): An update (2014–2018). *Clin Neurophysiol.* 2020;131(2):474–528.

Moisset X, Bouhassira D, Avez Couturier J, et al. Pharmacological and non-pharmacological treatments for neuropathic pain: Systematic review and French recommendations. *Rev Neurol.* 2020;176(5):325–352.

Quesada C, Pommier B, Fauchon C, et al. New procedure of high-frequency repetitive transcranial magnetic stimulation for central neuropathic pain: A placebo-controlled randomized crossover study. *Pain.* 2020;161(4):718–728.

42 When Do I Refer for Invasive Therapies?

Nadine Attal and Didier Bouhassira

A 60-year-old man with a past history of repeated sciatica from disc herniations suffered a major car accident on the highway 2 years ago. This caused cauda equina syndrome with paraplegia and sensory loss. Since then, he has suffered from extremely severe pain paroxysms described as innumerable electric shocks. He has not responded to gabapentin, pregabalin, duloxetine, venlafaxine, oxcarbazepine, nortriptyline, iv ketamine, and transcutaneous electrical nerve stimulation. He recently received oxycodone (up to 80 mg per day), which had insufficient efficacy and caused somnolence. Smoked cannabis has transient effects on his pain paroxysms, but he avoids smoking every day. Complementary techniques (e.g., hypnosis) and psychotherapy are not beneficial. He is otherwise in good health, practices sport (swimming), is married, and has a 10-year-old son, but he has not yet been able to resume his past professional activity because of the pain. He is not depressed nor particularly anxious, but he cannot tolerate his pain anymore.

What do you do now?

This man suffers from severe paroxysmal neuropathic pain totally or partially refractory to first-, second-, and third-line pharmacological treatments. He is otherwise in good health, does not present with psychological or psychiatric comorbidity, has resumed his work despite his pain and paraplegia, and is extremely motivated. Long-term use of strong doses of opioids in this patient is detrimental for his professional activity and places him at risk of abuse. For this patient, invasive therapy may be discussed, and opioids should be progressively tapered off subsequently.

Invasive therapies for neuropathic pain should only be considered after multidisciplinary evaluation (Table 42.1). Best candidates are those with regional neuropathic pain (these therapies should be avoided for patients with diffuse pain because of the possibility of amplification phenomena, except if the pain results from a cervical spinal lesion) when

TABLE 42.1 **Main Indications for the Most Commonly Proposed Invasive Therapies in Neuropathic Pain**

Nature of Invasive Therapy	Neuropathic Pain Conditions
Peripheral nerve stimulation or dorsal root ganglion stimulation	Peripheral neuropathic pain preferably involving a nerve trunk (e.g., postsurgical nerve lesion)
Spinal cord stimulation	Failed back surgery syndrome Painful sensory neuropathy, particularly diabetic polyneuropathy (more evidence)
Epidural motor cortex or deep brain stimulation	Peripheral or central neuropathic pain refractory to all conventional therapies
Intrathecal therapy (ziconotide, morphine)	Peripheral or central neuropathic pain refractory to all conventional therapies preferably involving the lower limbs
DREzotomy	Brachial or lumbar plexus avulsion (with paroxysmal pain) with severe sensorimotor deficit Cauda equina syndrome (with paroxysmal pain) with severe sensorimotor deficit
Gasser thermocoagulation	Trigeminal neuralgia

more conservative first- and second-line therapies have failed. Whether invasive therapies should be considered after or before a trial of strong opioids (third-line treatments for neuropathic pain) is debatable, and many invasive neurostimulation techniques may be recommended before trying opioids. Patients should always be carefully selected on the basis of a psychological evaluation and be aware of the short- and long-term benefits and potential risks of invasive therapies. Generally, the presence of active unstable psychosis, severe personality disorders, ongoing addiction, or severe ongoing depression is regarded as a contraindication for invasive techniques. However, if depression results solely from pain, this may be discussed with psychiatrists. The use of high doses of opioids for pain before surgery is not necessarily a contraindication, but patients with long-term use might develop tolerance and dependence and are at higher risk of chronic postsurgical pain; therefore, doses should be reduced to a minimum, if possible, because of surgery. In any case, invasive techniques may also largely contribute to the reduction or stoppage of opioid use. Finally, it is preferable to propose invasive therapies once chronic neuropathic pain is fully stabilized—that is, generally at least 12 months after onset. Conversely, such therapies should not be too much delayed to avoid severe psychological or psychiatric complications that may occur, particularly if pain is severe and long-lasting. The nature of invasive therapies depends on the clinical context, the origin of pain (peripheral or central), and the area of pain, and it should always be evidence based. By far the most commonly proposed and documented invasive therapies for neuropathic pain, outside the specific case of advanced cancer and palliative care, are spinal cord stimulation and related techniques. Other invasive techniques include mainly peripheral nerve stimulation or pulsed radiofrequency (which are minimally invasive), deep brain/epidural motor cortex stimulation, intrathecal therapy, and ablation surgery techniques in select conditions (Gasser thermocoagulation for idiopathic or classical trigeminal neuralgia; dorsal root entry zone [DREZ] for most severe cases of plexus avulsion or cauda equina syndrome). Other ablation surgical techniques, such as cordotomy or plexus neurolysis, may be proposed only in conditions of neuropathic and/or nociceptive pains associated with advanced refractory cancer and palliative care.

In this patient who suffers from severe refractory paroxysmal pain related to cauda equina syndrome with total sensory deafferentation of the painful legs, spinal cord and peripheral nerve stimulation are not appropriate because of his total sensory loss and risk of inefficacy. Conditional invasive treatments for this case (to be discussed with him after full multidisciplinary assessment, and psychiatric and psychological assessment) are intrathecal analgesic therapy, deep brain/epidural motor cortex stimulation, or DREZ (which consists of lesioning the entry zone of the roots). After full multidisciplinary assessment, the patient received intrathecal therapy at a specialized center, with morphine gradually increased from 0.1 to 1 mg per day. After 3 months, he reports 40% pain improvement and improvement in quality of life, with side effects mainly consisting of somnolence and fatigue. He has been able to gradually stop oral oxycodone.

KEY POINTS TO REMEMBER

· Invasive therapies for refractory neuropathic pain should be considered after multidisciplinary evaluation and include central or peripheral invasive neuromodulation techniques, intrathecal drug treatment, and ablative surgical techniques.
· Whether invasive therapies should be considered after or before a trial of strong opioids (third-line treatments for neuropathic pain) is debatable.
· Patients should be carefully selected on the basis of a psychological evaluation and be aware of the short- and long-term benefits and potential risks of these techniques.
· It is preferable to propose invasive therapies once chronic neuropathic pain is fully stabilized—that is, generally at least 12 months after onset.

Further Reading

Aichaoui F, Mertens P, Sindou M. Dorsal root entry zone lesioning for pain after brachial plexus avulsion: Results with special emphasis on differential effects on the paroxysmal versus the continuous components. A prospective study in a 29-patient consecutive series. *Pain.* 2011;152(8):1923–1930.

Gebreyohanes AMH, Ahmed AI, Choi D. Dorsal root entry zone lesioning for brachial plexus avulsion: A comprehensive literature review. *Oper Neurosurg.* 2021;20(4):324–333.

Knotkova H, Hamani C, Sivanesan E, et al. Neuromodulation for chronic pain. *Lancet.* 2021;397(10289):2111–2124.

Moisset X, Bouhassira D, Avez Couturier J, et al. Pharmacological and non-pharmacological treatments for neuropathic pain: Systematic review and French recommendations. *Rev Neurol.* 2020;176(5):325–352.

43 Peripheral Nerve Stimulation and Pulsed Radiofrequency

Nadine Attal and Didier Bouhassira

A 56-year-old woman with rheumatoid arthritis suffers from pain radiating from the cervical region up to the eye, described as lightning, electric shocks, lancinating, and occurring at least 10 times per day. Pain is triggered by any cervical movement. At examination, there is radiating pain induced by pressure at the upper cervical region. The rest of the neurological examination is normal. She has not tolerated several antineuropathic drugs, including gabapentin, pregabalin, duloxetine, and amitriptyline. Two C2–C3 anesthetic nerve blocks conducted in 6-month intervals totally relieved her pain, but it returned after a few months.

What do you do now?

This woman reports paroxysmal pain (electric shocks) radiating from the cervical region up to the eye corresponding to the territory of the occipital nerve. The pain area, quality of pain, and the fact that it is triggered by cervical movements and increased by pressure at the upper cervical region orient toward occipital neuralgia. Occipital neuralgia is characterized by severe, paroxysmal, shooting or stabbing pain in the distribution of the greater occipital, lesser occipital, and/or third occipital nerves. Although it is classified as headache, it may be considered neuropathic because it is caused by compression of the occipital nerve generally due to arthritis or antlantoaxoidal osteoarthritis. Other etiologies mainly include trauma, cervical cord tumor, and Chiari malformation. The management of occipital neuralgia includes antineuropathic drugs, nerve blocks, and surgical interventions. Diagnosis was here confirmed by ultrasound-guided somatic nerve block with local anesthetics of C2–C3.

Because this woman has occipital neuralgia and was refractory to conservative treatment including nerve blocks and antineuropathic drugs, she appears to be a good candidate for more invasive approaches, which include mainly peripheral nerve stimulation (PNS) and, to a lesser extent, pulsed radiofrequency.

This woman received two anesthetic nerve occipital blocks with good, albeit transient, efficacy. After a successful PNS trialing, psychological assessment, and multidisciplinary concertation, she was treated by implanted occipital nerve stimulation 2 years ago and has remained largely alleviated since then.

Peripheral nerve stimulation commonly uses percutaneously placed devices consisting of an implantable electrode, a microprocessor receiver, and a pulse generator. The best indication is peripheral neuropathic pain affecting one or two nerve territories (although most studies have limitations and blinding is questionable). Occipital nerve stimulation (Figure 43.1) has been mainly studied in occipital neuralgia (with positive results based on generally low-quality studies), migraine, and cluster headache. Side effects mainly include electrode migrations (10–20%) and, less commonly, habituation or tolerance, infection, cutaneous erosions, local pain, or muscle spasms.

Pulsed radiofrequency works by delivering a targeted electrical field to the dorsal root ganglion via a catheter needle tip, without causing damage

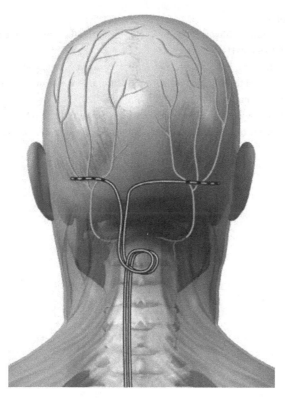

FIGURE 43.1 Occipital nerve stimulation.

because the temperature is maintained below 42°C. A few randomized controlled trials have showed the efficacy of pulsed radiofrequency in thoracic postherpetic neuralgia and in cervical radiculopathy.

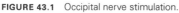

KEY POINTS TO REMEMBER

- The best potential indication for peripheral nerve stimulation is refractory peripheral neuropathic pain involving one nerve territory, although the level of evidence for efficacy remains low.
- Pulsed radiofrequency may be best proposed for refractory patients with thoracic postherpetic neuralgia or cervical radiculopathy with a moderate quality of evidence.

Further Reading

Knotkova H, Hamani C, Sivanesan E, et al. Neuromodulation for chronic pain. *Lancet*. 2021;397(10289):2111–2124.

Moisset X, Bouhassira D, Avez Couturier J, et al. Pharmacological and non-pharmacological treatments for neuropathic pain: Systematic review and French recommendations. *Rev Neurol*. 2020;176(5):325–352.

Wu CY, Lin HC, Chen SF, et al. Efficacy of pulsed radiofrequency in herpetic neuralgia: A meta-analysis of randomized controlled trials. *Clin J Pain*. 2020;36(11):887–895.

44 Spinal Cord Stimulation

Nadine Attal and Didier Bouhassira

A 48-year-old farmer without relevant medical
history suffers from chronic low back and left leg
pain despite surgery for discal herniation 2 years
ago. His low back pain is mild to moderate. His
leg pain covers the posterior part of the left thigh
and leg up to the plantar surface and toe. It is
described as electric shocks and burning, and it is
rated 7/10 on a 0–10 NRS. He has not responded
to several well-conducted treatments, including
nonsteroidal anti-inflammatory drugs, epidural
infiltrations, gabapentin, pregabalin, duloxetine,
and physiotherapy. Transcutaneous electrical nerve
stimulation is partially effective but has limited post
effect (1 hour) and is judged difficult to use every
day. He does not wish to receive strong opioids
because his brother died from drug addiction. He has
sleep problems but is not depressed. He is currently
treated with tramadol paracetamol six pills per day
with poor efficacy (10%). Electromyography (EMG)
confirms chronic sciatic left S1 radiculopathy.

What do you do now?

This man suffers from chronic back and leg pain despite spinal surgery, also called failed back surgery syndrome (FBSS). This generally corresponds to mixed pain because pain at the lower back is mostly nociceptive, whereas pain at the leg generally corresponds to neuropathic pain (the more extended the leg pain to the distal part of the foot, the more neuropathic). In this patient, only leg pain was neuropathic, situated in a neuroanatomical area (i.e., left S1 dermatoma), with confirmation of the radicular lesion by EMG. It did not respond to first- and second-line medications, and he was reluctant to receive strong opioids. He was oriented to a specialist for conventional spinal cord stimulation (SCS).

Spinal cord stimulation uses a device that delivers electrical stimuli to the spinal cord (Figures 44.1 and 44.2). It has been mainly studied in three neuropathic pain indications: FBSS (it is more effective for neuropathic leg pain than back pain), complex regional pain syndrome, and diabetic painful neuropathy. Contraindications include pacemaker or cardiac defibrillator (this requires a cardiologist's advice before the procedure), severe thrombocytopenia, uncontrolled coagulopathy, active infection, and unstable psychosis (but not major depression or anxiety

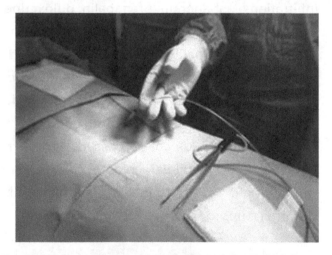

FIGURE 44.1 Percutaneous implantation of electrodes for spinal cord stimulation.

Source: Provided with courtesy from Sophie Colnat and Phillippe Rigoard (France).

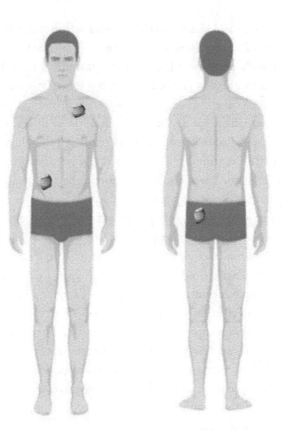

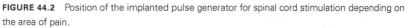

FIGURE 44.2 Position of the implanted pulse generator for spinal cord stimulation depending on the area of pain.

Source: Provided with courtesy by Sophie Colnat and Phillippe Rigoard (France).

syndromes, which are often related to pain). Decisions should be taken after pluriprofessional assessment, including psychologist or psychiatrist advice, to ensure that the patient is clearly aware and has no fear of the technique.

This patient was a good candidate for SCS: He had FBSS with predominantly neuropathic pain, refractory to well-conducted first- and second-line treatments, pain was well circumscribed, he had no contraindications, and he was fully aware of the benefits and risks of the techniques. After giving consent to surgery and receiving appropriate information, he received a trial period of 10 days, as generally recommended: The surgeon implanted a temporary device and inserted the electrodes in the epidural space of the spine (Figure 44.2). After 10 days, the patient experienced 70% pain relief. He then received a permanent implantation procedure, with the generator placed underneath the skin (at the buttock, but it may also be the lower abdomen), and the trial electrodes were replaced with sterile electrodes. This was done as outpatient surgery, and he was allowed to leave the hospital once the anesthesia had worn off. He was authorized to return to work and drive again (with the stimulator turned off) 1 week after surgery. Because the material implanted was not ferromagnetic, he has no limitations for further magnetic resonance imaging.

There is a large consensus that pain relief with conventional SCS is associated with paresthesias covering the area of pain and that mechanisms are hence related to activation of large myelinated (Aβ) fibers by the electrical stimulation, based on the classical gate theory of pain (also proposed for transcutaneous electrical nerve stimulation, Chapter 33). However, SCS may have other mechanisms; it may reinforce GABAergic inhibition in the spinal cord and act on supraspinal mechanisms. Frequency of stimulation ranges between 20 and 120 Hz. Adverse events are rare (<15% of cases) and mostly include lead migration or breakage and infection. SCS may be best implanted percutaneously, which allows peroperative testing of pain relief, or surgically for patients with past spinal surgery (this allows to stimulate a larger area with surgical electrodes).

Newer SCS technologies include high- to very high-frequency stimulations (10,000 Hz) of generally short duration and low amplitude, which do not induce paresthesia (and thus make it possible to conduct double-blind studies); burst stimulation (pulse trains of consecutive waves); closed-loop SCS (which allow to adjust and optimize the stimulation current); and dorsal root ganglion stimulation (for pain in the distribution of dorsal to sacral dermatomas [i.e., T10 to S2]). Complications are rare, related to hardware dysfunction (migration, disconnection, and electrode breakage) and implant site pain. The risk of spinal cord damage (through epidural hematoma) is extremely low. Dorsal root ganglion stimulation seems to be associated with higher risk of lead migration and damage than SCS.

- Among implantable neurostimulation techniques for neuropathic pain, conventional SCS has been the most widely used.
- SCS is currently recommended for peripheral neuropathic pain due to radiculopathy (FBSS), diabetic neuropathy (painful diabetic neuropathy), and complex regional pain syndrome.
- Newer techniques include high- to very high-frequency SCS, dorsal root stimulation, and burst SCS.

Further Reading

Attal N, Perrot S, Fermanian J, Bouhassira D. The neuropathic components of chronic low back pain: A prospective multicenter study using the DN4 questionnaire. *J Pain*. 2011;12:1080–1087.

Cruccu G, Garcia-Larrea L, Hansson P, et al. EAN guidelines on central neurostimulation therapy in chronic pain conditions. *Eur J Neurol*. 2016;23:1489–1499.

Knotkova H, Hamani C, Sivanesan E, et al. Neuromodulation for chronic pain. *Lancet*. 2021;397:2111–2124.

Mekhail N, Levy RM, Deer TR et al Evoke Study Group. Long-term safety and efficacy of closed-loop spinal cord stimulation to treat chronic back and leg pain (Evoke): a double-blind, randomised, controlled trial. *Lancet Neurol*. 2020 Feb;19(2):123–134.

Petersen EA, Stauss TG, Scowcroft JA et al. Effect of High-frequency (10-kHz) Spinal Cord Stimulation in Patients With Painful Diabetic Neuropathy: A Randomized Clinical Trial. *JAMA Neurol*. 2021;78:687–698.

45 Invasive Brain Stimulation and Intrathecal Therapy

Nadine Attal and Didier Bouhassira

A 52-year-old policeman had a severe horse riding accident responsible for spinal cord injury (T10 level). Since then, he has partially recovered his motor function, but suffers from severe neuropathic pain, involving inferior limbs and the abdomen up to T10 level. Pain is described as burning, squeezing, and sensitive to touch. He also has bladder dysfunction and constipation. Examination discloses tactile and thermoalgesic hypoesthesia at the lower limbs and evoked pain to brush at level. Drug treatments including duloxetine and gabapentin are ineffective, whereas strong opioids, tramadol and amitriptyline, were stopped because of dysuria and constipation. He has been receiving pregabalin for more than 2 years, but he has recently increased the dosage up to 600 mg per day because of decreased efficacy over time and now reports multiple side effects. Furthermore, when he forgets his treatment, he feels an urge to take his pill. Spinal cord stimulation is disregarded because of the lesion of the spinal cord.

What do you do now?

This patient has traumatic spinal cord injury responsible for at-level allodynia and below-level spontaneous pain. He is refractory to first-, second-, and third-line medications and seems to be dependent on pregabalin. Hence, invasive treatments may be considered. Because spinal cord stimulation is difficult in this case due to spinal cord lesion, therapeutic options include mainly intrathecal analgesics or invasive brain stimulation. Noninvasive brain stimulation such as repetitive transcranial magnetic stimulation might have been proposed, but the patient has no access to this treatment, which is conducted in very limited centers.

After careful psychological assessment and multidisciplinary concertation meeting, it was decided to propose intrathecal therapy. Intrathecal pain therapy involves implanting a catheter into the cerebrospinal fluid, which is then connected to an intrathecal pump implanted under the skin of the patient's abdomen (Figure 45.1). Three drugs are labeled by the U.S. Food and Drug Administration for intrathecal administration: morphine, ziconotide, and baclofen. Intrathecal therapy for chronic noncancer pain may also use clonidine or local anesthetics, but only morphine and ziconotide have been assessed in prospective randomized controlled studies

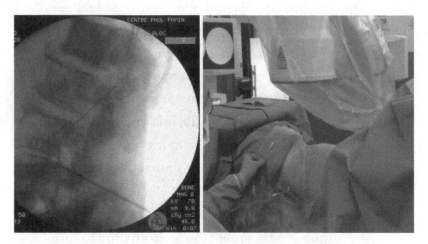

FIGURE 45.1 Intrathecal therapy. The implantation is generally conducted under general anesthesia under radiological guidance control to guide the position of the catheter in the intrathecal space in the spine. The pump is generally implanted in the lower quadrant of the abdominal region.

Photographs provided by Denis Dupoiron (Centre Paul Papin, Angers, France).

for chronic refractory pain (although none have been specifically assessed in neuropathic pain). Most common side effects of intrathecal morphine are nausea/vomiting, urinary retention, and pruritus, whereas serious complications include catheter granulomas, respiratory depression, tolerance, and dependence. Trialing and small initial dosages are recommended. Ziconotide is a synthetic compound of the ω-conopeptide derived from the *Conus magus* fish (it is a potent selective N-type channel blocker and blocks central neurotransmission). It can only be administered intrathecally because of poor blood–brain barrier penetration and a high risk of hypotension. It has many side effects (9 patients out of 10), including nausea and central nervous system effects (dizziness, nystagmus, memory impairment, somnolence, asthenia, headache, blurred vision, and confusion); the worst is psychosis. For these reasons, the decision to use ziconotide for chronic noncancer pain should be made after careful multidisciplinary assessment, including psychological and psychiatric evaluation; the drug is contraindicated in patients with past or current psychosis. Due to a narrow therapeutic window, ziconotide requires careful dose titration.

The patient was first treated by intrathecal morphine (up to 0.8 mg/day), but this treatment had to be stopped because of urinary retention and pruritus (which is more frequent with intrathecal morphine than with oral morphine). With the lack of psychiatric contraindication, ziconotide (Prialt, 100 µg/ml) was introduced at low initial dosages (2.4 µg/day) and was slowly titrated by 2 µg every 48 hours until a dose of 8 µg/day was obtained. This dosage seemed to be fairly tolerated and reduced pain by more than 70%. After 3 months, the patient reports 50% pain improvement and improvement in quality of life, with side effects mainly consisting of somnolence and fatigue. After 6 months of maintenance therapy, side effects are insignificant. Although pain improvement is now less consistent (30% pain relief), the patient has remained satisfied with the treatment and has been able to stop pregabalin.

Motor cortex stimulation (MCS) involves the placement of electrodes along the surface of the brain in the precentral gyrus, corresponding to the motor cortex area (Figure 45.2). Mechanisms may involve activation of the endogenous opioid systems. It has been suggested that a good selection of patients (particularly those responding to noninvasive brain stimulation [i.e., rTMS of the motor cortex]) might enhance its efficacy. A recent

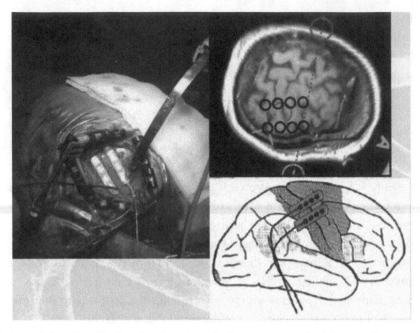

FIGURE 45.2   Site of implantation of the electrodes for motor cortex stimulation upon the precentral gyrus.

Reproduced with permission from JP Lefaucheur and JP Nguyen.

small (albeit high-quality) double-blind placebo-controlled crossover trial in 18 patients with severe refractory neuropathic pain suggested that approximately 40% responded to MCS, particularly those with facial pain, phantom limb pain, and complex regional pain syndrome. Deep brain stimulation (several potential targets) may act through autonomic mechanisms or endogenous opioids. Despite long-standing use, its level of evidence for intractable neuropathic pain remains inconclusive. Therefore, this therapy is very seldom proposed and generally not recommended.

KEY POINTS TO REMEMBER

- Intrathecal therapy and brain invasive neurostimulation, particularly epidural motor cortex stimulation, may be considered for very refractory patients with neuropathic pain

after careful multidisciplinary concertation and psychological assessment.
- Recent high-quality studies suggest the efficacy of motor cortex stimulation in refractory neuropathic pain.

Further Reading

Brookes ME, Eldabe S, Batterham A. Ziconotide monotherapy: A systematic review of randomised controlled trials. *Curr Neuropharmacol*. 2017;15(2):217–231.

Cruccu G, Garcia-Larrea L, Hansson P, et al. EAN guidelines on central neurostimulation therapy in chronic pain conditions. *Eur J Neurol*. 2016;23:1489–1499.

Deer TR, Pope JE, Hanes MC, McDowell GC. Intrathecal therapy for chronic pain: A review of morphine and ziconotide as firstline options. *Pain Med*. 2019;20(4):784–798.

Hamani C, Fonoff ET, Parravano DC, et al. Motor cortex stimulation for chronic neuropathic pain: Results of a double-blind randomized study. *Brain*. 2021;144(10):2994–3004.

Knotkova H, Hamani C, Sivanesan E, et al. Neuromodulation for chronic pain. *Lancet*. 2021;397:2111–2124.

Moisset X, Bouhassira D, Avez Couturier J, et al. Pharmacological and non-pharmacological treatments for neuropathic pain: Systematic review and French recommendations. *Rev Neurol*. 2020;176:325–352.

Index